DEVELOPING AND SUSTAINING AN EFFECTIVE AND RESILIENT ONCOLOGY CAREFORCE

PROCEEDINGS OF A WORKSHOP

Erin Balogh, Emily Zevon, Margie Patlak, and
Sharyl J. Nass, *Rapporteurs*

National Cancer Policy Forum

Board on Health Care Services

Health and Medicine Division

The National Academies of
SCIENCES · ENGINEERING · MEDICINE

THE NATIONAL ACADEMIES PRESS
Washington, DC
www.nap.edu

THE NATIONAL ACADEMIES PRESS   500 Fifth Street, NW   Washington, DC 20001

This activity was supported by Contract No. 200-2011-38807 (Task Order No. 75D30118F00071) and Contract No. HHSN263201800029I (Task Order No. HHSN26300008) with the Centers for Disease Control and Prevention and the National Cancer Institute/National Institutes of Health, respectively, and by the American Association for Cancer Research, American Cancer Society, American College of Radiology, American Society of Clinical Oncology, Association of American Cancer Institutes, Association of Community Cancer Centers, Bristol-Myers Squibb, Cancer Support Community, CEO Roundtable on Cancer, Flatiron Health, Helsinn Therapeutics (U.S.), Inc., LIVESTRONG Foundation, Merck, National Comprehensive Cancer Network, Novartis Oncology, Oncology Nursing Society, and Pfizer Inc. Any opinions, findings, conclusions, or recommendations expressed in this publication do not necessarily reflect the views of any organization or agency that provided support for the project.

International Standard Book Number-13: 978-0-309-49604-9
International Standard Book Number-10: 0-309-49604-7
Digital Object Identifier: https://doi.org/10.17226/25533

Additional copies of this publication are available from the National Academies Press, 500 Fifth Street, NW, Keck 360, Washington, DC 20001; (800) 624-6242 or (202) 334-3313; http://www.nap.edu.

Printed in the United States of America

Suggested citation: National Academies of Sciences, Engineering, and Medicine. 2019. *Developing and sustaining an effective and resilient oncology careforce: Proceedings of a workshop.* Washington, DC: The National Academies Press. https://doi.org/10.17226/25533.

The National Academies of
SCIENCES · ENGINEERING · MEDICINE

The **National Academy of Sciences** was established in 1863 by an Act of Congress, signed by President Lincoln, as a private, nongovernmental institution to advise the nation on issues related to science and technology. Members are elected by their peers for outstanding contributions to research. Dr. Marcia McNutt is president.

The **National Academy of Engineering** was established in 1964 under the charter of the National Academy of Sciences to bring the practices of engineering to advising the nation. Members are elected by their peers for extraordinary contributions to engineering. Dr. John L. Anderson is president.

The **National Academy of Medicine** (formerly the Institute of Medicine) was established in 1970 under the charter of the National Academy of Sciences to advise the nation on medical and health issues. Members are elected by their peers for distinguished contributions to medicine and health. Dr. Victor J. Dzau is president.

The three Academies work together as the **National Academies of Sciences, Engineering, and Medicine** to provide independent, objective analysis and advice to the nation and conduct other activities to solve complex problems and inform public policy decisions. The National Academies also encourage education and research, recognize outstanding contributions to knowledge, and increase public understanding in matters of science, engineering, and medicine.

Learn more about the National Academies of Sciences, Engineering, and Medicine at **www.nationalacademies.org**.

The National Academies of
SCIENCES · ENGINEERING · MEDICINE

Consensus Study Reports published by the National Academies of Sciences, Engineering, and Medicine document the evidence-based consensus on the study's statement of task by an authoring committee of experts. Reports typically include findings, conclusions, and recommendations based on information gathered by the committee and the committee's deliberations. Each report has been subjected to a rigorous and independent peer-review process and it represents the position of the National Academies on the statement of task.

Proceedings published by the National Academies of Sciences, Engineering, and Medicine chronicle the presentations and discussions at a workshop, symposium, or other event convened by the National Academies. The statements and opinions contained in proceedings are those of the participants and are not endorsed by other participants, the planning committee, or the National Academies.

For information about other products and activities of the National Academies, please visit www.nationalacademies.org/about/whatwedo.

WORKSHOP PLANNING COMMITTEE[1]

LISA KENNEDY SHELDON (*Co-Chair*), Chief Clinical Officer, Oncology Nursing Society

LAWRENCE N. SHULMAN (*Co-Chair*), Professor of Medicine, Deputy Director for Clinical Services, and Director, Center for Global Cancer Medicine, Abramson Cancer Center, University of Pennsylvania

AMY P. ABERNETHY, Chief Medical Officer, Chief Scientific Officer, and Senior Vice President, Oncology, Flatiron Health[2]

EDWARD J. BENZ, JR., President and Chief Executive Officer Emeritus, Dana-Farber Cancer Institute; Richard and Susan Smith Distinguished Professor of Medicine, Genetics and Pediatrics, Harvard Medical School

ROBERT W. CARLSON, Chief Executive Officer, National Comprehensive Cancer Network

CLESE ERIKSON, Deputy Director, Health Workforce Research Center, The George Washington University

STANTON L. GERSON, Director, Case Comprehensive Cancer Center, Professor of Hematological Oncology; Case Western Reserve University; Director, University Hospitals Seidman Cancer Center

LORI HOFFMAN HÕGG, Veterans Health Administration National Program Manager, Prevention Policy, National Center for Health Promotion and Disease Prevention; National Oncology Clinical Advisor, Office of Nursing Services, Department of Veterans Affairs

RUTH E. NEMIRE, President, ASK Educational Games, LLC

RANDALL A. OYER, Medical Director, Oncology, Ann B. Barshinger Cancer Institute, Penn Medicine Lancaster General Health

DAVID SIEGEL, LCDR, U.S. Public Health Service, Centers for Disease Control and Prevention, National Center for Chronic Disease Prevention and Health Promotion, Division of Cancer Prevention and Control, Epidemiology and Applied Research Branch

---

[1] The National Academies of Sciences, Engineering, and Medicine's planning committees are solely responsible for organizing the workshop, identifying topics, and choosing speakers. The responsibility for the published Proceedings of a Workshop rests with the workshop rapporteurs and the institution.

[2] As of February 2019, Dr. Abernethy's affiliation is Principal Deputy Commissioner and Acting Chief Information Officer of Food and Drugs, Food and Drug Administration.

VIRGINIA L. VALENTIN, Assistant Professor and Associate Director, Division of Physician Assistant Studies, Department of Family and Preventive Medicine, University of Utah School of Medicine

ROBERT A. WINN, Associate Vice Chancellor, Community-Based Practice; Professor of Medicine, Division of Pulmonary and Critical Care Medicine, University of Illinois at Chicago; Director, University of Illinois Cancer Center

Project Staff

ERIN BALOGH, Senior Program Officer
RUTH COOPER, Senior Program Assistant
ANNALEE GONZALES, Administrative Assistant
EMILY ZEVON, Associate Program Officer
SHARYL J. NASS, Forum Director and Director, Board on Health Care Services

NATIONAL CANCER POLICY FORUM[1]

EDWARD J. BENZ, JR. (*Chair*), President and Chief Executive Officer Emeritus, Dana-Farber Cancer Institute; Richard and Susan Smith Distinguished Professor of Medicine, Genetics and Pediatrics, Harvard Medical School

GARNET L. ANDERSON, Senior Vice President and Director, Public Health Sciences Division, Fred Hutchinson Cancer Research Center; Affiliate Professor, Department of Biostatistics, University of Washington

KENNETH ANDERSON, Kraft Family Professor of Medicine, American Cancer Society Clinical Research Director, Jerome Lipper Multiple Myeloma Center, Harvard Medical School, Dana-Farber Cancer Institute

WILLIAM L. BAILEY, Vice President, Medical & Scientific Affairs Research & Development, Helsinn Therapeutics (U.S.), Inc.

KAREN BASEN-ENGQUIST, Annie Laurie Howard Research Distinguished Professor, Professor of Behavioral Science, and Director, Center for Energy Balance in Cancer Prevention and Survivorship, The University of Texas MD Anderson Cancer Center

CHRIS BOSHOFF, Chief Development Officer, Oncology, Global Product Development, Pfizer Inc.

CATHY J. BRADLEY, Associate Dean for Research, Colorado School of Public Health, Professor and Deputy Director, University of Colorado Cancer Center

OTIS W. BRAWLEY, Bloomberg Distinguished Professor, Department of Epidemiology, Bloomberg School of Public Health, Department of Oncology, School of Medicine, Johns Hopkins University

ROBERT W. CARLSON, Chief Executive Officer, National Comprehensive Cancer Network

---

[1] The National Academies of Sciences, Engineering, and Medicine's forums and roundtables do not issue, review, or approve individual documents. The responsibility for the published Proceedings of a Workshop rests with the workshop rapporteurs and the institution.

NANCY E. DAVIDSON, President and Executive Director, Seattle Cancer Care Alliance; Senior Vice President, Director, and Full Member, Clinical Research Division, Fred Hutchinson Cancer Research Center; Head, Department of Medicine, Division of Medical Oncology, University of Washington

GEORGE D. DEMETRI, Professor of Medicine and Director, Ludwig Center, Harvard Medical School; Senior Vice President for Experimental Therapeutics, Dana-Farber Cancer Institute; Associate Director for Clinical Sciences, Dana-Farber/Harvard Cancer Center

JAMES H. DOROSHOW, Deputy Director for Clinical and Translational Research, National Cancer Institute

NICOLE F. DOWLING, Associate Director for Science, Division of Cancer Prevention and Control, Centers for Disease Control and Prevention

SCOT W. EBBINGHAUS, Vice President and Therapeutic Area Head, Oncology Clinical Research, Merck Research Laboratories

KOJO S. J. ELENITOBA-JOHNSON, Professor, Perelman School of Medicine; Director, Center for Personalized Diagnostics and Division of Precision and Computational Diagnostics, University of Pennsylvania

AWNY FARAJALLAH, Vice President, Head, US Medical Oncology, Bristol-Myers Squibb

STANTON L. GERSON, Director, Case Comprehensive Cancer Center; Professor of Hematological Oncology; Case Western Reserve University; Director, University Hospitals Seidman Cancer Center

LORI HOFFMAN HŌGG, Veterans Health Administration National Program Manager, Prevention Policy, National Center for Health Promotion and Disease Prevention; National Oncology Clinical Advisor, Office of Nursing Services, Department of Veterans Affairs

LINDA HOUSE, President, Cancer Support Community

HEDVIG HRICAK, Chair, Department of Radiology, Memorial Sloan Kettering Cancer Center

ROY A. JENSEN, President, Association of American Cancer Institutes; Director, The University of Kansas Cancer Center; William R. Jewell, M.D. Distinguished Masonic Professor, Kansas Masonic Cancer Research Institute

LISA KENNEDY SHELDON, Chief Clinical Officer, Oncology Nursing Society

SAMIR N. KHLEIF, Director, Jeannie and Tony Loop Immuno-Oncology Lab, Biomedical Scholar and Professor of Oncology, Georgetown Lombardi Comprehensive Cancer Center, Georgetown University Medical Center

RONALD M. KLINE, Medical Officer, Patient Care Models Group, Center for Medicare & Medicaid Innovation, Centers for Medicare & Medicaid Services

MICHELLE M. LE BEAU, Arthur and Marian Edelstein Professor of Medicine and Director, The University of Chicago Comprehensive Cancer Center

MIA LEVY, Director, Rush University Cancer Center; Associate Professor of Medicine, Division of Hematology and Oncology; System Vice President, Cancer Services, Rush System for Health

J. LEONARD LICHTENFELD, Interim Chief Medical Officer, American Cancer Society

NEAL J. MEROPOL, Vice President, Research Oncology, Flatiron Health

MARTIN J. MURPHY, Chief Executive Officer, CEO Roundtable on Cancer

RANDALL A. OYER, Medical Director, Oncology, Ann B. Barshinger Cancer Institute, Penn Medicine Lancaster General Health

RICHARD PAZDUR, Director, Oncology Center of Excellence; Acting Director, Office of Hematology and Oncology Products, Food and Drug Administration

RICHARD L. SCHILSKY, Senior Vice President and Chief Medical Officer, American Society of Clinical Oncology

DEBORAH SCHRAG, Chief, Division of Population Sciences, Professor of Medicine, Department of Medical Oncology, Harvard Medical School, Dana-Farber Cancer Institute

LAWRENCE N. SHULMAN, Professor of Medicine, Deputy Director for Clinical Services, and Director, Center for Global Cancer Medicine, Abramson Cancer Center, University of Pennsylvania

DAN THEODORESCU, Director, Samuel Oschin Comprehensive Cancer Institute, Cedars-Sinai Medical Center

VERENA VOELTER, Head, United States Oncology Clinical Development & Medical Affairs, Novartis Pharmaceuticals Corporation

GEORGE J. WEINER, C.E. Block Chair of Cancer Research, Professor of Internal Medicine, and Director, Holden Comprehensive Cancer Center, The University of Iowa

ROBERT A. WINN, Associate Vice Chancellor, Community-Based Practice; Professor of Medicine, Division of Pulmonary and Critical Care Medicine, University of Illinois at Chicago; Director, University of Illinois Cancer Center

National Cancer Policy Forum Staff

ERIN BALOGH, Senior Program Officer
RUTH COOPER, Senior Program Assistant
ANNALEE GONZALES, Administrative Assistant
NATALIE LUBIN, Research Assistant
MICAH WINOGRAD, Financial Officer
EMILY ZEVON, Associate Program Officer
SHARYL J. NASS, Forum Director and Director, Board on Health Care Services

Reviewers

This Proceedings of a Workshop was read in draft form by Lauren Shern and Taryn Young within the National Academies of Sciences, Engineering, and Medicine to ensure the proceedings meets institutional standards for quality and objectivity while accurately reflecting the purpose and focus of the workshop.

Acknowledgments

Support from the many annual sponsors of the National Academies of Sciences, Engineering, and Medicine's National Cancer Policy Forum is crucial to the work of the forum. Federal sponsors include the Centers for Disease Control and Prevention and the National Cancer Institute/National Institutes of Health. Non-federal sponsors include the American Association for Cancer Research, American Cancer Society, American College of Radiology, American Society of Clinical Oncology, Association of American Cancer Institutes, Association of Community Cancer Centers, Bristol-Myers Squibb, Cancer Support Community, CEO Roundtable on Cancer, Flatiron Health, Helsinn Therapeutics (U.S.), Inc., LIVESTRONG Foundation, Merck, National Comprehensive Cancer Network, Novartis Oncology, Oncology Nursing Society, and Pfizer Inc.

The forum wishes to express its gratitude to the expert speakers whose presentations helped further the dialogue and advance progress to better support the oncology careforce and improve the delivery of high-quality cancer care. The forum also wishes to thank the members of the planning committee for their work in developing an excellent workshop agenda.

Contents

Boxes and Figures

BOXES

FIGURES

Acronyms and Abbreviations

ACA	Patient Protection and Affordable Care Act
ACCC	Association of Community Cancer Centers
AMA	American Medical Association
AMIA	American Medical Informatics Association
APP	advanced practice provider
ASCO	American Society of Clinical Oncology
CEO	chief executive officer
CMS	Centers for Medicare & Medicaid Services
CSC	Cancer Support Community
EHR	electronic health record
FDA	Food and Drug Administration
HPV	human papillomavirus
IOM	Institute of Medicine
NP	nurse practitioner

OMH Oncology Medical Home
ONS Oncology Nursing Society

PA physician assistant
PCORI Patient-Centered Outcomes Research Institute
PTSD posttraumatic stress disorder

SCH Symptom Care at Home

VA Department of Veterans Affairs
VHA Veterans Health Administration

Proceedings of a Workshop

WORKSHOP OVERVIEW[1]

The landscape of cancer care is undergoing rapid change. While the age-adjusted mortality rate from cancer is declining, population growth and the aging of the U.S. population are contributing to increases in the number of patients diagnosed with cancer. Advances in cancer research, screening and diagnostic practices, and cancer treatment have led to improved outcomes for patients with cancer and a growing population of cancer survivors, but those factors have also increased the complexity of cancer care. The overall number of cancer survivors—both those undergoing active treatment and those who have completed treatment—is increasing more rapidly than the number of clinicians available to care for them, raising concern about the U.S. health care system's capacity to deliver high-quality cancer care in the coming years (IOM, 2013a). Other factors affecting the delivery of cancer care include the introduction of new payment models that increase clinician accountability for the value of cancer care; a growing emphasis on interprofessional, collaborative practice; and the widespread adoption of technologies in clinical practice with variable levels of usability, efficiency, and clinician burden (e.g., electronic

---

[1] The planning committee's role was limited to planning the workshop, and the Proceedings of a Workshop was prepared by the workshop rapporteurs as a factual summary of what occurred at the workshop. Statements, recommendations, and opinions expressed are those of the individual presenters and participants, and are not necessarily endorsed or verified by the National Academies of Sciences, Engineering, and Medicine, and they should not be construed as reflecting any group consensus.

1

health records [EHRs]) (Burwell, 2015; NASEM, 2015, 2018a; Ommaya et al., 2018). The provision of cancer care has also shifted primarily to the outpatient setting, in which patients and family caregivers shoulder more responsibilities related to cancer treatment and recovery (NASEM, 2016).

These trends in cancer care are having a major impact on the oncology careforce—defined in this workshop proceedings as the spectrum of health care professionals caring for patients with cancer (e.g., physicians, advanced practice providers, nurses, pharmacists, and other clinicians) along with family caregivers. To examine opportunities to better support the oncology careforce and improve the delivery of high-quality cancer care, the National Cancer Policy Forum held a workshop on Developing and Sustaining an Effective and Resilient Oncology Careforce on February 11–12, 2019, in Washington, DC. The workshop convened stakeholders with a broad range of expertise, including clinicians and representatives of health professional societies, health care organizations and oncology practices, insurers, and federal agencies, as well as patients and patient advocates.

The workshop included presentations and panel discussions on:

- Trends in demographics, the careforce, and oncology practice, and the implications for the future of cancer care;
- Strategies to improve the organization and delivery of cancer care; and
- Opportunities to change policy and leverage technologies in oncology care.

This Proceedings of a Workshop highlights suggestions from individual participants to enhance the delivery of high-quality patient care by improving the development and support of the oncology careforce. These suggestions are discussed throughout the proceedings and are summarized in Box 1. Appendix A includes the Statement of Task for the workshop. The workshop agenda is provided in Appendix B. Speakers' presentations and the webcast have been archived online.[2]

---

[2] See http://www.nationalacademies.org/hmd/Activities/Disease/NCPF/2019-FEB-11. aspx (accessed May 17, 2019).

BOX 1
Suggestions from Individual Workshop Participants to Enhance the Delivery of High-Quality Patient Care by Improving the Development and Support of the Oncology Careforce

Improving Careforce Training, Accreditation, and Licensure
- Provide clinical informatics training for clinicians. (Sesto)
- Offer oncology training for physician assistants (PAs) and nurse practitioners (NPs) via fellowships, residency, or other post-graduate structured curriculum to enable more autonomous practice. (Hyde)
- Promote partnerships with health professional organizations to enhance teaching, educational programs, and demonstration projects. (Van Houtven)
- Provide training in communications and health literacy. (Back, Portman, Scroggins, Van Houtven)
- Provide earlier educational opportunities in oncology and cancer prevention. (Brawley, Nevidjon, Shulman, Winn)
- Provide patient navigation training to PAs, NPs, nurses, pharmacists, and other cancer clinicians. (Nemire)
- Provide undergraduate, graduate, and continuing education in palliative care for all cancer care professionals as well as patients. (Hyde, Portman, Scroggins)
- Create a national licensure system for clinicians that states could opt into, to facilitate the practice of telemedicine across state lines. (Dentzer, Dillon, Hyde, Nemire)

Reducing Administrative Burdens by Improving the Design and Usability of Electronic Health Records (EHRs)
- Incorporate improved clinical usability in EHR certification requirements. (Back)
- Design EHRs so patient data are readily accessible. (Shulman)
- Improve EHR design elements, such as text boxes that are too small to fully display text as well as requirements for redundant documentation. (Sesto)
- Standardize quality measures in EHRs and make them easier to report. (Paz, Sesto)
- Identify clinical trial candidates through EHRs and collect follow-up data within the record. (Meropol)

continued

BOX 1 Continued

Prioritizing Research to Improve Cancer Care
- Evaluate the effectiveness of innovative models of care delivery, including their impact on managing new treatments, technologies, and programs. (Bruinooge, Cox, Levy, Shulman)
- Determine the optimal treatment regimens for cancer therapies to shorten treatment duration and discontinue ineffective treatments. (Morris, Oyer, Van Houtven)
- Integrate implementation science and collaborate with diverse organizations to enhance adoption of research findings. (Birken, Van Houtven)

Implementing Innovative Payment Models
- Identify innovative models and best practices for alternative payment models. (Shulman)
- Implement reimbursement models that enable more autonomous practice of PAs and NPs. (Hyde)
- Move away from fee-for-service reimbursement and toward value-based reimbursement models. (Lichtenfeld, Mooney, Paz, Shipman)
- Develop new payment models to support greater use of telemedicine. (Dentzer)
- Offer financial incentives for health care providers to implement effective innovations in care. (Mooney)

Using Innovative Technologies, Tools, and Strategies to Support the Cancer Careforce
- Create user-friendly technologies for clinicians, patients, and caregivers. (Lichtenfeld, Mooney, Shulman)
- Make technologies available on smartphones, the Internet, and other devices that clinicians and patients rely on and are more inclined to use. (Mooney, Shulman)
- Design technologies that can be easily tailored to the specific needs of patients or health care settings. (Mooney)
- Include common standard elements, including usability across different patient populations and transparency around underlying digital coding and algorithms. (Dentzer)
- Predicate all technologies on interoperability, seamless data and information exchange, and data accessibility with appropriate privacy and security safeguards. (Dentzer)

- Create a public–private initiative to help health care systems acquire and implement the most clinically and cost-effective technologies. (Dentzer)
- Develop a national plan for universal, affordable, high-speed broadband access to help reduce health disparities. (Dentzer, Lichtenfeld, Winn)

Leveraging Organizational Culture and Leadership to Promote Clinician Well-Being
- Build teams structured on a foundation of dignity, respect, shared accountability, and core organizational values. (Back, Carlson, Cox, Levy)
- Foster careforce well-being through interventions such as mindfulness training and well-being self-assessments with national benchmarks. (Back)
- Institute policies to improve the clinical work environment, including measurement of clinician satisfaction, incentives for collaboration and teamwork, and opportunities for renewal that are integrated into clinician workflow. (Back)
- Establish formal mentoring programs for clinicians. (Carlson, Nevidjon)
- Encourage collaboration among professional societies to address clinician burnout. (Morris, Nevidjon, Oyer)

Improving Partnerships Between Specialties and Promoting Multidisciplinary Teams
- Facilitate partnerships between oncology clinicians and primary care physicians. (Jacobs, Scroggins, Shulman)
- Extend the capacity of cancer care teams by increasing the autonomy and roles of NPs, PAs, and pharmacists in patient navigation, treatment, follow-up care, and palliative care. (Högg, Nemire, Portman)
- Reduce practice inefficiencies through improved care delivery models that enhance coordination among care team members. (Van Houtven)
- Facilitate interprofessional education and implement standards for training interdisciplinary health care teams. (Nevidjon, Van Houtven)
- Provide funding and staff for palliative care services and program certification, and include palliative care parameters in reported quality metrics. (Portman)
- Coordinate with hospice and other community-based care providers to expand patient access to services. (Portman)

continued

BOX 1 Continued

Including Caregivers in the Care Team and Alleviating Caregiving Burdens
- Integrate caregivers into the cancer care team. (Bruinooge, Scroggins, Van Houtven)
- Assess and reinforce caregivers' skills via training programs. (Portman, Van Houtven)
- Ask patients what role they would like their caregivers to have during the first visit. (Bruinooge, Van Houtven)
- Consult with caregivers on patient symptoms and preferences through "virtual huddles." (Van Houtven)
- Use digital tools to more effectively involve and integrate caregivers on the care team. (Portman)
- Increase access to home care provided by professional nurses and nurse aides. (Dentzer)
- Provide paid family leave or tax credits for family caregivers. (Van Houtven)
- Make home- and community-based care a standard health insurance benefit, and adopt lifetime patient cost caps on insurance. (Van Houtven)
- Offer remote patient monitoring and clinical visits to relieve transportation and time burdens through emerging technologies. (Dentzer, Levy, Portman, Takvorian)

CANCER CARE TRENDS AND CAREFORCE NEEDS

Many workshop participants described how different factors are influencing the landscape of cancer care, such as

- cancer incidence and prevalence, including inequities in cancer risk and outcomes;
- capacity, distribution, and well-being of the cancer careforce; and
- changes in the delivery of cancer care, including the growing complexity of care, greater reliance on family caregiving, increased use of technology, and payment and delivery system reforms.

Promoting Patient-Centered Care
- Integrate oncology navigators into the care team and involve them from the point of diagnosis. (Burris, Cantril, Rosenthal, Scroggins)
- Consider patient experiences in workplace design. (Cantril, Shulman)
- Imbed cancer care in multidisciplinary care clinics alongside cardiology, diabetes, and other specialty care for easier and more efficient patient access. (Bruinooge)
- Offer group visits with clinicians, particularly in survivorship care. (Bruinooge)
- Offer suburban satellite care to relieve the transportation burden and inconvenience for patients who live far from urban cancer centers. (Burris, Jacobs)
- Coordinate scheduling to enable all follow-up care in one visit. (Jacobs)
- Address patient well-being via real-time symptom reports that are integrated into the EHR and offer shared decision making. (Portman)
- Screen patients regularly for their palliative care needs. (Portman, Scroggins)
- Partner with corporate community partners to reduce barriers to patient care. (Cantril, Dillon, Levy, Scroggins)

Epidemiological Trends in Cancer

Otis Brawley, Bloomberg Distinguished Professor at Johns Hopkins University, provided an overview of the epidemiological trends that project an increased demand for cancer care.

He noted that although the age-adjusted cancer mortality rate has declined 27 percent in the past two decades (Siegel et al., 2018), the number of patients diagnosed with cancer in the United States is predicted to rise from 1.8 million in 2019 to 2.3 million in 2035 (AACR, 2018). The number of cancer survivors is also expected to rise from 15.5 million in 2016 to 20.3 million in 2026 (ACS, 2016).

Brawley noted that these increases are due to a growing and aging population, changes in screening and diagnostic practices, and changes in population risk. Between 2005 and 2050, the nation's population will increase from 296 million to 438 million, a growth of 48 percent (Passel and Cohn, 2008). At the same time, the U.S. population is aging, and cancer is more prevalent among older adults—the median age of cancer diagnosis is 65 years in women and 66 years in men (Siegel et al., 2018). Smoking, overweight/obesity, and a lack of physical activity are the biggest modifiable risk factors for the development of cancer (IOM, 2013b; NASEM, 2018b). Although smoking-related cancers are continuing to decline, Brawley noted that excess caloric intake and insufficient exercise are likely to become the leading causes of cancer in the United States in the near future. Two-thirds of adults and one-third of children are currently overweight or obese, and cancers associated with overweight and obesity are expected to increase 30 to 40 percent between 2010 and 2020 (Weir et al., 2015a). The incidence of cancers associated with viral infections are also projected to rise within this decade: liver cancer incidence is expected to increase by 50 percent due to hepatitis B and C infections, and oral cancers in white men are expected to increase by 30 percent due to infection with human papillomavirus (HPV) (Weir et al., 2015a,b). Given these changes in population risk, Brawley stressed that "prevention of cancer is clearly a need in the future." He cited one study estimating that cancer deaths could be reduced by more than 50 percent if all known modifiable risk factors were addressed via preventive measures (Colditz et al., 2012).[3]

Brawley noted that even though population-wide mortality rates have declined, cancer care disparities remain a persistent problem. For example, Brawley reported that there are significant disparities in breast, prostate, and colorectal cancer mortality between black and white Americans, and these disparities have worsened since the 1970s (Siegel et al., 2018) (see Figure 1). He stressed that access to cancer care is unevenly distributed among population subgroups. Thus, as cancer screening, diagnostic, and treatment approaches become more effective, these improvements could exacerbate disparities by race and ethnicity, socioeconomic status, and geography. In terms of geography, Brawley highlighted state-based disparities in cancer risk and mortality. He noted that since 1980, age-adjusted colorectal cancer mortality has declined by 50 percent nationwide, but in Louisiana and Mississippi, colorectal cancer mortality has declined by only 12 percent (Siegel et al., 2018). There are similar state-based disparities in breast and lung cancer mortality (Siegel et al., 2018). Some of the lung cancer disparities can be attributed to a higher prevalence of behavioral risk factors; states with the highest rates of lung cancer are also those with the highest prevalence of smoking (CDC, 2018). Brawley added that there are disparities in cancer outcomes based on educational achievement. Americans with a college degree are less likely to die from cancer than Americans without a college degree; if all Americans had the cancer mor-

---

[3] The National Cancer Policy Forum is planning a 2020–2021 workshop series to examine opportunities for improving cancer prevention, risk reduction, and screening.

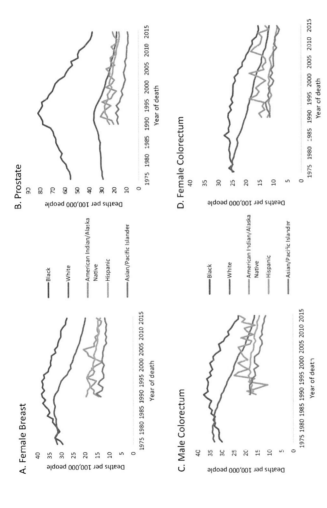

FIGURE 1 Cancer mortality in breast, prostate, and colorectal cancer from 1990 to 2015 by race/ethnicity. Death rates are illustrated for (A) breast cancer (female), (B) prostate cancer, (C) colorectal cancer (male), and (D) colorectal cancer (female).
NOTES: Rates are per 100,000 and age-adjusted to the 2000 U.S. standard population. Rates for American Indians/Alaska Natives (AIs/ANs) are based on the Contract Health Service Delivery Area counties. Rates for Hispanics exclude Louisiana, New Hampshire, and Oklahoma. Rates for whites, blacks, Asians/Pacific Islanders, and AIs/ANs are not exclusive of Hispanic origin. Data source: National Center for Health Statistics.
SOURCES: Brawley presentation, February 11, 2019; Siegel et al., 2018.

tality rate of college-educated Americans, Brawley said 150,000 deaths from cancer would be averted this year (Siegel et al., 2018).

Disparities in cancer outcomes may also result from poor access to cancer care. Suanna Bruinooge, director of the research strategy and operations division of the American Society of Clinical Oncology (ASCO), noted that 43 percent of patients with cancer experienced barriers to accessing optimal cancer care due to inadequate health insurance (ASCO, 2018).

Workforce Projections

Bruinooge said the growing number of cancer survivors and the aging of the U.S. population are projected to outpace the oncology workforce. She pointed to an ASCO workforce study that predicted a 48 percent increase in demand for oncology services between 2005 and 2020, but only a 14 percent increase in the number of oncologists (Erikson et al., 2007). A more recent workforce study was consistent with the earlier study, but concluded that the shortages may occur later than previously predicted and that the Patient Protection and Affordable Care Act (ACA) may modestly exacerbate the oncology workforce shortage (Yang et al., 2014). Bruinooge added that aging of the oncology workforce is a key contributor to this mismatch: "We have a lot of people nearing retirement, and we don't have as many people coming up to replace them," she said. Another factor that may be contributing to the shortage of oncologists is that fewer medical residents are selecting oncology as a specialty, said Anthony Back, professor and co-director of the Cambia Palliative Care Center of Excellence at the University of Washington. He cited a study that found residents reported being less likely to pursue a career in oncology after they completed a hematology/oncology rotation (McFarland et al., 2015). Back also noted from personal experience that medical residents often express dissatisfaction with oncology rotations, reporting that they feel like "order monkeys" whose sole function is to enter treatment orders dictated by attending physicians.

Workshop participants noted that the aging oncology workforce will also create a shortage of oncology nurses. Brenda Nevidjon, chief executive officer (CEO) of the Oncology Nursing Society (ONS) and professor at Duke University, said the average age of nurses currently in practice is 50 (McDonnell, 2017). Nevidjon noted that baby boomer nurses are retiring, and estimated that more than 1 million nurses will retire between 2019 and 2030. Although there has been nationwide expansion in nursing school enrollment, "We're losing an accumulated knowledge and clinical expertise base with a shift toward younger nurses. All of us are going to be challenged with how to retain some of that expertise and coach and mentor younger nurses," Nevidjon said. She added that it often takes 1 year for new nurses to gain the skills and experience necessary to function effectively in clinical settings, and that it is unrealistic to expect nursing staff to be fully functional after a typical 4- to 6-week orientation.

Nevidjon noted that nurses with experience and specialty training in oncology are increasingly rare. In a nationwide 2017 survey, only 2.8 percent of responding registered nurses identified oncology as their specialty (Smiley et al., 2018). In a 2017 survey of community cancer centers, 60 percent of responding institutions reported a shortage of oncology nurses (ACCC, 2017). Nevidjon also noted that national changes in nurse practitioner (NP) education have resulted in fewer oncology concentrations, requiring NPs interested in oncology to seek additional training after completion of their degree.

Distribution of the Workforce

Additionally, Bruinooge and Nevidjon pointed to the uneven nationwide distribution of oncology clinicians and cancer care facilities. Bruinooge reported that oncology practices are concentrated in areas with large populations of older adults and are also clustered around academic medical centers (Kirkwood et al., 2018) (see Figure 2). A nationwide ASCO survey of patients with cancer found that rural patients spend 66 percent more time traveling to receive oncology care than patients living in non-rural areas (ASCO, 2018).

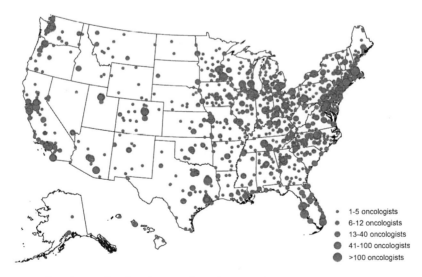

FIGURE 2 Geographic distribution of oncology practices.
SOURCE: Bruinooge presentation, February 11, 2019; reprinted by permission from ASCO.

Nevidjon noted that nursing resources are also unevenly distributed across the country; some states, including Florida and Ohio, are projected to have a surplus of nurses, while others, including California and Texas, are projected to have a shortage (HHS et al., 2017). David Morris, radiation oncologist at SSM Health Medical Group, noted that there are also geographic disparities in the availability of radiation oncology facilities. Brawley added that a recent study found that in many areas in the United States, a patient would have to travel a great distance to access a radiation therapy facility (Ballas et al., 2006). He noted that there are also geographic disparities in access to pathology services.

Clinician Burnout

A number of speakers described the role that burnout can play in attrition among the oncology workforce. Clinician burnout is defined as a syndrome of emotional exhaustion, depersonalization, and reduced feeling of personal accomplishment (Maslach and Jackson, 1981). Nevidjon said nursing burnout is related to work overload; conflicting values; a lack of control, reward, or fairness in the workplace; and a missing sense of community. She added that nurses may also experience compassion fatigue, which results from ongoing exposure to pain and suffering. She said that addressing burnout and compassion fatigue requires both system-level changes as well as self-care interventions for individual clinicians.

Randall Oyer, medical director of the Ann B. Barshinger Cancer Institute of Penn Medicine Lancaster General Health, stressed that burnout can be exacerbated by the perception that a person's work is not valuable. "No matter how many patients we have, if we know we are making a difference … it gets us through the day and gives us some satisfaction. We need to figure out ways to remove the work that is not meaningful," he said. Nevidjon reported that a recent American Medical Association (AMA) survey found that physicians and their staff spent, on average, approximately 15 hours per week obtaining insurance pre-authorizations for patients (AMA, 2018). Nurses and physicians who feel they are wasting their energy on administrative tasks may be more inclined to retire early from a cancer care career, Nevidjon added. Mark Hyde, director of advanced practice care at the Huntsman Cancer Institute and professor at The University of Utah, referred to data from the American Academy of Physician Assistants indicating that approximately 30 percent of physician assistants (PAs) report feelings of burnout, with the highest prevalence of burnout occurring between the fifth and ninth year of practice (AAPA, 2018). Hyde noted that this high frequency of burnout, and the subsequent loss of qualified clinicians, is at significant cost to health care systems.

Back agreed that clinician burnout has increased, and suggested that this trend can partly be attributed to the burden of using EHRs, particularly the extra time required for data entry and retrieval. He discussed a study that found physicians who used EHRs and computerized order entry experienced higher rates of burnout (Shanafelt et al., 2016). Leigh Boehmer, medical director of education for the Association of Community Cancer Centers (ACCC), reported that in an ACCC member survey, two-thirds of respondents reported that they felt "a great deal of stress" from their job and only one-quarter reported that they had sufficient time to complete required clinical documentation. Lawrence Shulman, deputy director for clinical services at the Abramson Cancer Center of the University of Pennsylvania, added that EHRs and the documentation they require have become more taxing as cancer care has become more complex. "It's harder to find what we need in the EHR to provide the best care," he said.

Mary Sesto, an associate professor in the Department of Medicine at the University of Wisconsin–Madison, agreed, noting that many clinicians spend as much time using EHRs as they spend on patient care. Compared with physicians in other countries, American physicians provide more documentation per outpatient visit (Downing et al., 2018) (see Figure 3). Referring to this phenomenon as "note bloat," Sesto quoted from Downing et al. (2018): "The highly trained U.S. physician has become a data-entry clerk, required to document not only diagnoses, physician orders, and patient visit notes, but also an increasing amount of low-value administrative data." Mia Levy, director of the Rush University Cancer Center, noted that the large volume of emails and text messages to which clinicians have to respond adds to this administrative burden, as does time spent digitally accessing health care information on patients seen at other facilities. "It really is overwhelming when we think about how much data we are creating as part of our health care system, as well as the number of emails and text messages we are getting every day, and the different ways we interface with all of the systems involved in our patients' care," she said.

Workshop participants noted that an additional factor contributing to clinician burnout is the high cost of cancer care and the associated burden to patients and health care systems. Harold Paz, executive vice president and chief medical officer of Aetna, noted that most cancer drugs launched between 2009 and 2014 were priced at more than $100,000 per patient per year of treatment, with recently approved drugs costing more than $400,000 per patient per year (President's Cancer Panel, 2018). John Cox, medical director of oncology services at Parkland Health System of the University of Texas Southwestern Medical Center, noted that financial considerations often affect patient care because many patients lack sufficient insurance. The high cost of treatment also contributes to the time clinicians have to spend obtaining preauthorizations. "The workforce is very dispirited when you deal with that day in and day out," Cox said.

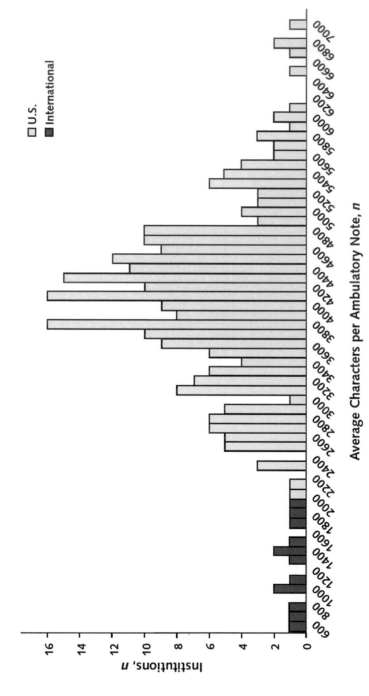

FIGURE 3 Documentation volume for outpatient visits in the United States compared with other countries.
SOURCES: Sesto presentation, February 12, 2019; reproduced from Downing et al., 2018.

Complex and Time-Consuming Cancer Care

Several workshop speakers discussed the complexity of contemporary cancer care, noting that it can require more frequent patient visits and more clinician time devoted to diagnosis and treatment. "The work effort is not just directly related to the number of cancer patients, but has to do with the new prolonged and complex therapies. Every patient diagnosed today is going to generate more work than they used to," Shulman said. For example, he said the new immunotherapies for cancer treatment can have serious side effects that require enhanced monitoring and management. Shulman cited data from an academic medical center demonstrating that between 2001 and 2007, the number of clinic visits devoted to new cancer patients increased by 23 percent, while the number of visits devoted to continuing patients increased by 93 percent (Shulman et al., 2009). He said that more recent data from academic medical center clinics that treat patients with breast or lung cancer demonstrate that the total number of patient and office visits have increased, even though the rate of new patient visits has not changed.[4]

Eben Rosenthal, Ann and John Doerr Medical Director of the Stanford Comprehensive Cancer Center, added that new targeted therapies and their associated molecular diagnostics have increased the complexity of cancer care. Levy pointed to the recent increase in data-based cancer care as an additional source of complexity. "We are getting a huge amount of data from other places that we were not getting even a few years ago," she said. Cynthia Cantril, director of cancer support services and patient navigation at Sutter Pacific Medical Foundation, agreed, noting that oncology clinicians are increasingly overloaded with data. "It is hard for us to keep up," she said.

Caregiving at Home

Lisa Kennedy Sheldon, chief clinical officer of ONS, noted that caregivers who provide support for patients with cancer are essential members of the oncology careforce. Courtney Harold Van Houtven, research scientist at the Durham Veterans Affairs Medical Center and professor at the Duke University School of Medicine, defined cancer caregivers as "family members or friends, typically uncompensated and providing care at home, who devote significant time, energy, and costs to caring for an individual with cancer." A recent survey found that during a 1-year period, there were at least 2.8 million cancer caregivers in the United States. Of these caregivers, 60 percent do not have a college degree and 64 percent report a household income of less than $75,000 per year (National Alliance for Caregiving and the AARP Public Policy Insti-

---

[4] Personal communication from Lawrence Shulman, February 2019.

tute, 2015). Although most caregivers report little to no formal training in the tasks they perform, 72 percent assist with medical or nursing tasks, such as administering injections, tube feedings, and catheter and colostomy care (Mollica et al., 2017; National Alliance for Caregiving and the AARP Public Policy Institute, 2015; van Ryn et al., 2011).

Recent changes in cancer treatment have increased the level of care that is provided by informal caregivers. Samuel Takvorian, chief fellow of the division of hematology and oncology at the Perelman School of Medicine at the University of Pennsylvania, noted that cancer treatment is increasingly available in the form of oral medications that can be taken at home, rather than infusions that occur in a clinic (Greer et al., 2016; Zerillo et al., 2018). "That's great for our patients, but it also means they are shouldering a greater responsibility for side effect monitoring, symptom management, and medication adherence," he said. Much of this responsibility falls on patients' family caregivers.

Van Houtven noted that informal caregivers face a variety of stressors and challenges, including a lack of training, fragmentation of care, not feeling valued and included in the care team, and economic burden (NASEM, 2016; Rosland and Piette, 2010; Silliman et al., 1996; Wolff et al., 2016). She noted that more than 50 percent of cancer caregivers report high levels of stress (National Alliance for Caregiving and the AARP Public Policy Institute, 2015). Kathi Mooney, interim director of the population sciences program and co-leader of the cancer control and population sciences program at the Huntsman Cancer Institute at The University of Utah, added that more than three-quarters of family caregivers for patients receiving home hospice care report feelings of anxiety as well as fatigue, disturbed sleep, depressed mood, and interference with normal activities (Reblin et al., 2019). Van Houtven noted that a major source of caregiver stress is financial strain due to not being able to work or having to reduce hours of work, combined with medical and transportation costs (de Moor et al., 2017; Kamal et al., 2017; Van Houtven et al., 2010). She added that preliminary results from an ongoing study of caregivers of patients with advanced solid tumors indicate that caregivers' median out-of-pocket costs were $581 over 14 days. More than half of caregivers in the study reported that they were struggling financially, with 25 percent of caregivers reporting that they were in "serious financial trouble." To address this burden, Van Houtven suggested implementing interventions to support caregivers and mitigate financial consequences of caregiving.

For example, several workshop participants suggested strategies to reduce caregiver burden by offering additional support for patient home care. Susan Dentzer, visiting fellow at the Duke–Margolis Center for Health Policy, referred to the "hospital at home" model, which involves hospital-level care at home to individuals who might normally be admitted to acute inpatient units, but who may achieve better outcomes if they are cared for at home by a broad team of providers (Federman et al., 2018). Dentzer noted that there is already a precedent for oncology home care set by clinics that offer home infusions of intravenous cancer medications. Because some patients are admitted to hospitals for symptom management or complications relating to cancer treatment, it is possible that they could instead be "hospitalized" at home. Van Houtven suggested supporting caregivers with community-based services to help them in the demanding post-surgery and post-treatment phases. "We have a ridiculously high expectation that family members can provide incredibly complex care, when someone who is a trained clinician could do this in the home if patients had that benefit [covered by health insurance]. But most people can't afford home nursing care, or are not covered for that in the U.S. health care system," Van Houtven explained.

OPPORTUNITIES TO ADDRESS ONCOLOGY CAREFORCE CHALLENGES

Given the growing number of cancer survivors, ongoing changes to oncology care, and concerns about the well-being of the oncology careforce, a number of workshop participants discussed potential changes to improve cancer care delivery and better support the careforce. Paz stated, "To get a more sustainable cancer care model, there's a great deal of work to do and it's going to take collaboration across the entire health care system with involvement of all parties, but … it's an achievable goal." Much of the workshop was devoted to considering potential strategies, including

- Exploring organizational changes to delivering oncology care;
- Leveraging technologies to better support clinicians, patients, and families; and
- Pursuing policy changes to support high-quality cancer care.

Organizational Opportunities

Many workshop speakers stressed that cancer care requires a collaborative team of clinicians that work in tandem with the patient and caregivers across multiple disciplines. These disciplines may include medical, surgical, and radiation oncology; nursing; social work; pharmacy; palliative care; primary care; and public health. Cantril stressed that patients are the most important members of oncology care teams and should be central to any workplace organization plan. "We need to understand what the patients' needs are," she said. Shulman agreed, noting that it is important to consider patient experience in assessing the optimal organization of cancer care. Workshop speakers also stressed that cancer care teams need to coordinate with members of non-oncology specialties, such as cardiologists and primary care clinicians, as well as social service providers. Van Houtven noted that older patients often have multiple comorbidities that need to be addressed by diverse clinicians. "We need to traverse the oncology silo to include other specialties so we have more holistic care," she said. Bruinooge suggested that cancer care could be embedded in multidisciplinary care clinics alongside cardiology, diabetes, and other specialty care so that patients can be seen by various specialists in a single clinic visit. Sesto added that clinical informatics experts should also be included in oncology care teams, and noted that there are newly developed board certifications and fellowships in the field.

To improve patient experience and access to care, Linda Jacobs, director of the Cancer Survivorship Center of Excellence at the Abramson Cancer Center at the University of Pennsylvania, suggested that large cancer centers could offer suburban satellites to reduce transportation burden for patients who live far from urban areas. Additionally, she suggested scheduling coordinated follow-up visits to minimize patients' travel and time for clinic visits. Howard "Skip" Burris, president and chief medical officer of the Sarah Cannon Research Institute, agreed, noting, "We have to take care of patients in the communities where they live. The more we can do closer to home, the better patient satisfaction will be if that care is done with the quality and speed that is necessary."

Presenters described opportunities to better organize oncology care teams, build capacity for oncology care, and improve well-being of the cancer careforce. These included

- Fostering high-performing oncology teams;
- Including caregivers on the oncology care team;
- Expanding patient navigation services;
- Expanding care team capacity with advanced practice providers;
- Promoting clinician well-being and fostering a supportive work environment; and
- Partnering with community resources.

Workshop participants also discussed strategies for implementing workplace changes and examples of organizations that have successfully implemented novel cancer care programs.

Fostering High-Functioning Oncology Teams

Given the team-based nature of cancer care, several speakers discussed characteristics of high-functioning teams. Cox said effective teams are defined by four characteristics: they are externally and internally recognized as a team, they are committed to achieving an explicit shared goal, they allow team members to work interdependently to achieve objectives, and they engage in regular reflection to adapt their objectives and processes. Applying these team characteristics to the practice of oncology, Cox noted, "We have to shift our attitudes, have more self-reflection, particularly for physicians, to really realize how interdependent we are, if we're going to provide good quality care." All team members need to feel psychologically safe and empowered so they are comfortable offering constructive criticism and addressing conflict. Back added that psychological safety is frequently identified as an important component of high-performance teams (Edmondson, 1999). Van Houtven noted that with complex and multidisciplinary teams, it is important to delegate tasks, share knowledge, and understand which team members are responsible for particular aspects of patient care.

Robert Carlson, CEO of the National Comprehensive Cancer Network, characterized high-performance teams as having a shared vision, well-defined (but still flexible) roles and responsibilities, strong relationships and communication, mutual trust and respect, high emotional intelligence, and a shared leadership structure. Levy agreed that high-functioning teams treat each team member with dignity and respect, regardless of whether the team member is a clinician, patient, or caregiver. Carlson noted that high-performance teams are both more productive and more rewarding for their members (Banker et al., 1996; Castka et al., 2001). He said high-performance teams improve morale and facilitate talent retention because they allow team members to feel empowered and appreciated. In contrast, poorly functioning teams are associated with employee attrition and lack of commitment to their work (Porath, 2016; Porath and Pearson, 2013). "It's a huge drain on the performance of an organization," Carlson cautioned.

Several workshop speakers said that high-performing teams need to be developed and nurtured, and this requires identifying organizational core values and aligning expectations of behavior to facilitate a strong, positive workplace culture. Back, Carlson, and Cox emphasized that this process requires strong institutional leadership. Carlson noted that good leaders unite people around an exciting, aspirational vision, and create a practical strategic plan to achieve that vision. Effective leaders will attract, develop, and retain the best talent, and will enable ongoing innovation by revising their vision and strategy as needed, Carlson said (Ashkenas and Manville, 2018). He added that leaders also should set an example by being relentlessly self-critical about how they are behaving, addressing problems, and holding themselves to the same standards as they would hold others in the organization. Communication is also critical to good leadership, Carlson stressed, adding, "It's not a one-way street. It's not only communicating the vision, strategies, etc., but also listening intensely."

Including Caregivers on the Oncology Care Team

Bruinooge suggested that caregivers should be provided the opportunity to participate in the cancer care team. "If patients and their family caregivers aren't involved in their care discussions, they sometimes feel like they're being acted upon and not part of the team," she said. Mary Jackson Scroggins, founding partner of Pinky Hugs, added that caregivers involved in treatment discussions want clinicians to engage with them as equal participants in patient care. She called for a new paradigm in how clinicians approach care partners who are not health professionals, emphasizing that caregivers want to be involved in a meaningful way. She stated, "They don't want to simply be called when it's time for implementation, but to be a part of the treatment planning.... They serve a purpose that nobody else can serve."

Van Houtven also emphasized the importance of integrating caregivers in cancer care, and suggested that caregivers' skills should be assessed and reinforced with relevant training: "It is really important to understand the caregiver's capacity to safely provide care, as so much high-skilled care for infusions and oral cancer medicines are going into the home." She added that clinicians should consult with caregivers on an ongoing basis to assess their capacity to meet patients' needs. At their first visit, patients could be asked what role they want their caregivers to take in their cancer care, and the caregivers could be asked how they would like to be involved. "There are evidence-based ways to get these preferences from the start," Van Houtven said. She added that caregivers are an important source of information regarding patients' symptoms and preferences, and suggested that care managers could serve as a liaison between caregivers and oncology teams. This collaboration could be accomplished through "virtual huddles," which she noted are common in geriatric care (Van Houtven et al., 2019). "If the caregiver can't come in, it's a very efficient way during a team huddle to bring them in to understand their preferences and what is going on with the patient," she said.

Expanding Patient Navigation Services

Cantril emphasized that patient navigation services are vital because of the growing complexity of cancer care. Patients may experience fear and anxiety associated with cancer care, and often face both existential and logistical challenges. Cantril noted that patient navigators can reduce these challenges by helping patients in managing their cancer care. "Patients want to be helped and guided, and we need to shift to a culture of service to provide that guidance," Cantril noted, adding, "Oncology navigation needs to be recognized as part of the innovation solution to create high-value health care." Scroggins stressed that navigation services can be beneficial for every cancer patient, not just those challenged by a lack of resources. "It is not about poverty, and the process is not driven by zip code. Everybody deserves a navigator," she said. Cantril agreed, noting that navigation is a critical tool to support patients, caregivers, and clinicians. Burris stated that the nurse navigation program at the Sarah Cannon Research Institute "has yielded great benefits in terms of efficiencies, the patient experience, and the physician experience. It has been a huge key to our success in a number of areas."

Cantril noted that she views navigation as the "hub" of the "wheel of cancer care" (see Figure 4) because patient navigators serve as the central organizers for cancer care activities. She stressed that navigators should guide patients through all forms of care, including medical oncology, physical therapy, and mental health services. Cantril also noted that navigators should be involved in patient care from the earliest point of contact, usually the time of diagnosis. "Navigation will guide patients home, no matter where their end home is," Cantril said.

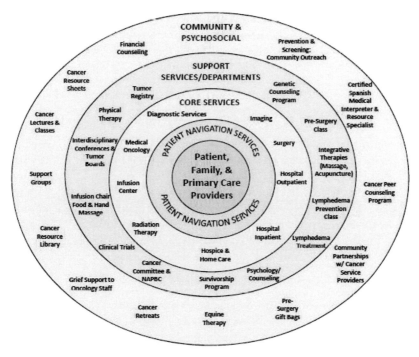

FIGURE 4 Patient navigation as the hub of the wheel of cancer care.
NOTE: NAPBC = National Accreditation Program for Breast Centers.
SOURCES: Cantril presentation, February 11, 2019; Reprinted with permission from Sutter Health.

Rosenthal noted that for navigation programs to function effectively, navigators need to be well integrated into the cancer care team. When he implemented a lay navigator program, he found that the separation of the navigator from the clinical care team made navigation less effective and led to duplication with social work efforts already in place. The navigation program became effective only after it was integrated into the care team so "the patient saw the navigator was not just somebody from the hospital helping with parking and directions, but part of their care team," Rosenthal said.

Integrating Palliative Care in Oncology Care

Many workshop participants described palliative care as an integral component of cancer care. Diane Portman, chair of the Supportive Care Medicine Department of the Moffitt Cancer Center and professor at the University of South Florida, defined palliative care as a person- and family-centered approach to care that provides relief from symptoms and stress of serious illness to improve quality of life for the patient and the family (NCP, 2018). Palliative care involves attending to the physical, functional, psychological, practical, and spiritual consequences of an illness, and can include assessment and management of patients' symptoms, assessment and support of caregiver needs, and planning and coordination of care. Portman stressed that palliative care is appropriate at any stage of a serious illness, and can be beneficial when provided with curative treatments as well as at the end of life (Ferrell et al., 2018).

Portman noted that palliative care resources are most effective when they are applied according to patients' needs and preferences. Palliative care involves working to identify what is most important to patients, families, and caregivers at every step in the process of cancer care. Portman said palliative care should attend holistically to patients' concerns and honor patients' perspectives, including the use of shared decision making to better align treatment based on patients' individual priorities. When patients are in remission, palliative care practitioners can continue to provide comfort care and help alert other clinicians to symptoms that may indicate recurrence or late effects of treatment.

Many types of clinicians provide palliative care, including nurses, NPs, physicians, PAs, chaplains, and social workers. "This care has to be team based because there is a lot of different expertise required to render the holistic care we must provide," Portman said. "Palliative care principles and practice can be delivered by clinicians caring for the oncology patients in any setting, not just by palliative care specialists," she stressed. Portman explained that she envisions palliative care as the fourth pillar of oncology care, along with radiation oncology, surgical oncology, and medical oncology, and encouraged all oncology clinicians to develop core palliative care competencies. While palliative care needs can often be managed by patients' primary oncology care team, some patients with complex symptoms may need high-level multidisciplinary care and specialist input or intensive care by a palliative care specialist. She suggested that clinicians should regularly screen patients for palliative care needs because needs may change over time as treatment continues or disease progresses. She noted that there are well-validated instruments available to conduct palliative care needs assessments (Waller et al., 2012).

Portman stressed the importance of health care leaders' support for palliative care. She suggested that this support may involve providing program funding and staff expansion for palliative care services, endorsing palliative program certification per national quality standards, and including palliative care parameters in reported quality metrics. Coordination with hospice and other community-based providers is also needed because not all palliative care is provided at cancer centers, she said.

Collaborating with Primary Care Clinicians for Cancer Survivorship Care

Some speakers at a previous Institute of Medicine (IOM) workshop suggested that follow-up care for many cancer survivors could be transitioned to primary care clinicians to mitigate the growing demand for cancer care services (IOM, 2009). However, Jacobs noted that some cancer survivors should continue to be seen by oncology specialists because of the risk of long-term complications or late effects of cancer treatments. She suggested that cancer survivors could be stratified by risk, with lower risk patients transitioned to primary care follow-up. However, she noted that many oncology clinicians are reluctant to discontinue follow-up with their patients, and patients may be reluctant to leave their oncology clinicians and transition to primary care clinicians. Nevidjon suggested that patients' reluctance to transition care may be partly due to a failure in communication; often patients are not told that their follow-up care could eventually be transitioned to their primary care clinicians. "Sometimes we don't set that expectation, so then patients become afraid of not staying connected," she said. Shulman added that transitioning oncology patients to primary care may also be challenging because primary care clinicians are also experiencing workforce shortages. He added that some primary care clinicians may not be equipped or have the bandwidth to care for cancer survivors with severe or long-term complications, and suggested supporting ongoing partnerships between oncology and primary care clinicians.

Bruinooge suggested that cancer survivors could participate in group visits with clinicians instead of traditional one-on-one clinic visits. Cantril noted that her cancer center offers a speaker series to address patients' post-cancer health and psychosocial concerns, including nutritional support, cognitive changes, sexuality, exercise, and advance care planning, all of which can be addressed in a group setting. These programs allow patients who have completed their treatment to remain connected with their cancer centers and receive support in a familiar environment without taxing cancer care resources. Scroggins noted that patients often feel vulnerable after treatment and may be anxious about cancer recurrence. Cantril responded that "a ripple effect of these programs is that patients feel less frightened after they complete their treatment."

Expanding Care Team Capacity with Advanced Practice Providers

Many workshop participants noted that oncology care team capacity could be expanded by increasing the clinical autonomy of NPs and PAs (i.e., advanced practice providers [APPs]) as well as pharmacists. Bruinooge said a survey of oncology practices found that 28 percent of APPs see patients independently, while 65 percent use a combined model in which they perform some visits independently and some in collaboration with a physician (Bruinooge et al., 2018). The same survey found that APPs who see patients independently see more patients than those who only see patients in combination with physicians. Bruinooge noted that although APPs often consult with oncologists, many maintain independent caseloads and run academic clinics when oncologists are absent. "Increasing access to care demands more clinicians working differently. As your oncology teams expand, they're going to be rich with NPs and PAs to extend quality oncology care," Cox said. Oyer suggested the solution entails not only having sufficient numbers of physicians, PAs, and NPs, but also in deploying them effectively. Hyde agreed, noting that the work of APPs often duplicates the work of oncologists during combined patient visits. He also said additional training is needed before APPs can practice independently. Jacobs noted previous calls for expanding the roles of NPs and PAs within team-based models for survivorship care (Erikson et al., 2007; IOM, 2006, 2009).

Ruth Nemire, associate executive vice president of the American Association of Colleges of Pharmacy, noted that another strategy to extend the capacity of cancer care teams is to support pharmacists to participate more fully in patient navigation, treatment, and palliative care. Lori Hoffman Högg, national oncology clinical advisor for the Office of Nursing Affairs of the Department of Veterans Affairs (VA), added that in some oncology settings, pharmacists are already extending capacity by independently running oral chemotherapy clinics. Portman noted that incorporating pharmacists as part of a palliative care team is a cost-effective strategy for expanding services (Lehn et al., 2018). "There are lots of ways to include pharmacists in the system as we rethink the careforce," Nemire noted.

Promoting Clinician Well-Being and Fostering a Supportive Work Environment

Back suggested that supporting the well-being of the oncology careforce requires actions at the levels of both the individual and the health care system. It is important to help clinicians develop skills that promote well-being and resilience, but it is also necessary to address policies and organizational factors that contribute to burnout and compassion fatigue. Back said an individual's resilience can be strengthened through energy management, mindful attention, identifying and maintaining healthy boundaries, reframing cognitive distortions (e.g., blaming one's self inappropriately for an undesired outcome), regulating emotions, and finding meaning in daily activities. He offered several examples of how institutions can help clinicians build these skills, including offering mindfulness training and programs that support mental health. Back also recommended frequent self-assessment, noting that clinicians often lack conscious awareness of their level of stress. He pointed to a study assessing the effect of an intensive educational program that included training in mindfulness, communication, and self-awareness, and noted that the intervention was associated with improvements in physician well-being and attitude (Krasner et al., 2009). "So there are things we can do, but you have to get physicians into a place where they are really ready to try some of this stuff," Back said. He also emphasized that it is the responsibility of health care organizations to offer opportunities for clinician renewal during the workday. "It is not the responsibility of clinicians to do this on their own, after they have been at work all day and then done their documentation for 2 to 3 hours at night," Back said.

Back noted that even clinicians with optimal resilience skills will not flourish in an unsupportive work environment. He noted that characteristics of a supportive work environment include optimized workload, enhanced efficiency, promotion of autonomy, work–life balance, upholding of values, and creation of community (Back et al., 2016). Back suggested that leadership is critical to promoting these positive workplace characteristics, citing a study from a large health care organization that found clinicians were less likely to experience burnout if their supervisors had strong leadership skills (Shanafelt et al., 2015). Back also suggested institutional and health care system policies to improve clinicians' work lives, including publicly reported measurements of clinician satisfaction and work characteristics, incentives and rewards for collaboration and teamwork, opportunities for clinician renewal that are integrated into clinician workflow, and new certification requirements for EHRs. Back noted that frustration with EHRs is a major source of clinician stress and frustration. Nevidjon agreed that burdensome EHRs, along with unnecessary administrative tasks associated with payment systems, often contribute to burnout. Strategies to improve EHRs are discussed in the Technology Opportunities section.

Reducing Administrative Burdens

Workshop participants discussed strategies for reducing administrative duties and health care practice inefficiencies that burden oncology clinicians. Paz spoke about Aetna's efforts to reduce clinician burden by streamlining data entry for health care quality metrics in EHRs. He noted a recent study indicating that physicians in four common specialties spent an average of 785 hours and $40,069 per physician each year reporting quality metrics (combined total of $15.4 billion) (Casalino et al., 2016). He noted the conclusion in a 2015 IOM consensus report that too many measures are in use, and that many available measures are not fit for purpose (IOM, 2015). "Quality measures are critical to ensuring safe and effective patient care, but in the current system, they cost too much in terms of human and financial capital," Paz stressed. He reported on Aetna's participation in the Core Quality Measures Collaborative,[5] which convenes leaders from the Centers for Medicare & Medicaid Services (CMS), the National Quality Forum, and national physician organizations to reduce and standardize quality measures entered into EHRs. This collaborative, composed of public and private stakeholders, promotes quality measure alignment and harmonization and seeks to reduce burden by eliminating low-value and redundant metrics. Paz reported that the collaborative recently released a core set of quality measures in key clinical areas, including oncology.

Shulman agreed and noted that EHR development was driven largely by billing requirements and other regulatory factors, and "not necessarily by optimal ways to provide efficient, safe, and effective care." He stressed that "all of us spend more time than we would like in preauthorization, documentation, and other administrative tasks. While there are reasons for why we've needed to do that, we need to look at what the downstream implications of that are—we're caring for fewer patients than we might have if we had a more efficient way to deal with these tasks."

Rosenthal described Stanford's efforts to reduce the EHR burden on clinicians through the use of scribes, or individuals who provide documentation assistance. Often recent college graduates aspiring to attend medical school, scribes are accepted to a 1-year fellowship during which they are trained to complete documentation during patient visits with clinicians. Rosenthal reported that the program has reduced the time physicians spend on the computer as well as the length of patient visits with medical oncologists, which has resulted in shorter patient wait times prior to appointments. Physicians reported satisfaction with the scribes, who enabled them to work more efficiently and spend less time reviewing and submitting orders. "Patients were

---

[5] For more information on the Core Quality Measures Collaborative, see https://www.healthaffairs.org/do/10.1377/hblog20150623.048730/full/#core (accessed July 19, 2019).

able to spend more time with their doctors, and overall, the physicians have routinely reported that their quality of life has improved," Rosenthal said. He suggested that scribes are most effective in high-volume practices that require more than six notes per session, and when they are consistently paired with the same clinicians. However, Rosenthal noted that the scribe program is an additional institutional cost and there is frequent scribe turnover. He also emphasized that despite the success of the scribe program, scribing is a short-term solution to clinician burden related to EHRs and does not address the fundamental problem of poor usability.

Another way to improve care efficiencies is to improve coordination of care among members of the treatment team, Shulman said. He noted at his institution, because medical oncologists cannot manage the large intake of new patients, some patients may be initially seen by radiation oncologists for the work-up and to initiate further evaluations, even if they ultimately are going to have systemic therapy rather than radiation. Morris pointed out that treatments can also be streamlined. He noted that research has shown that certain radiation therapy courses can be shortened without hampering their effectiveness, and that the University of Pittsburgh recently instituted a shortened course of radiation therapy for breast cancer patients at its cancer care facility. Van Houtven suggested that another way to improve practice efficiencies is to discontinue treatments no longer seen to be effective. Oyer agreed that it is "really important to stop doing things that don't matter, or have unproven or minimal benefit."

Partnering with Community Resources

Several workshop participants identified community resources to support patients' needs. These resources included patient support groups and organizations, hospice facilities, and businesses that can transport patients to appointments and deliver medical supplies.

Bruinooge noted that social isolation can be detrimental to patients' health and well-being, and emphasized the importance of strong support systems (Cacioppo and Cacioppo, 2014). She and other workshop participants suggested that cancer survivors can serve as a valuable source of support for patients currently undergoing treatment. Cantril described a program that pairs volunteers with newly diagnosed patients to offer companionship and social support. She noted that these volunteers function as an extension of the patient navigator program, and can help meets patients' needs in health care organizations with limited resources for psychosocial oncology care.

Hildy Dillon, senior vice president of education and support systems at the Cancer Support Community (CSC), suggested that community partnerships can be a powerful source of support for patients and families. While major cancer centers can offer psychosocial oncology services, smaller practices can draw on community resources to provide emotional support, counseling, and patient navigation services. "We have to think about creative partnerships in smaller communities where there is not the diversity of practitioners that you might have in a cancer center," Dillon said. Hōgg added, "I have seen the community take care of patients when the resources are not available or they do not have nearby access to a health care institution. We could learn from these low-resource areas about what is working well and apply it even into the high-resource areas where patients might be getting a lot of care, but not getting all the care they need and desire."

Cantril noted that her cancer center uses free or discounted services provided by Lyft™ and Airbnb™ to provide transportation and housing for patients who may otherwise face difficulties accessing care. She noted that cancer care teams and health care organizations need to use innovative strategies to broaden their community interface. Levy agreed that corporate community partners can play an important role in reducing barriers to patient care. Scroggins added, "The community steps up if they see you are providing a service." She noted that when her organization ran a health fair, more than 20 small businesses donated food and other goods, as well as money to support the event.

Implementing Workplace Changes

Workshop participants presented examples of programs at their institutions for creating a sustainable and resilient cancer careforce (see Box 2). However, several participants identified implementation challenges due to diverse institutional and human factors. Nevidjon noted, "People get comfortable with how they've done things, so resistance to change can be very strong."

To generate support for workplace improvements, Oyer suggested articulating a shared goal and outlining a clear plan for how and when the goal will be achieved. "We need measurements we can stick to and keep ourselves on task to make sure we are doing what we promised to do," he stated.

Shulman also stressed the importance of having a realistic implementation plan, noting that changes that challenge existing structures and practices are more likely to fail without careful and sound planning. Other workshop participants noted that more profound careforce improvements will require policy changes and reassessment of current practices. Suggested policy changes are discussed further in the Policy Opportunities section.

Van Houtven noted that it is important to be able to assess improvement to incentivize and reward team-based care. She suggested measuring employee satisfaction both as a performance metric and to better understand how a health care organization's policy and organizational changes affect employees

BOX 2
Examples of Careforce Models for
Cancer Care Programs and Organizations

University of Pennsylvania's Cancer Survivorship Program

Linda Jacobs, director of the Cancer Survivorship Center of Excellence at the Abramson Cancer Center of the University of Pennsylvania, described her institution's comprehensive program for cancer survivorship and follow-up care. The program integrates survivorship follow-up visits, referrals to primary care, patient education, and outcome evaluation. It is modeled on guidelines from the National Comprehensive Cancer Network, the American Cancer Society, and the American Society of Clinical Oncology. Patient care services are provided by advanced practice providers (APPs) who were involved with the patient's care during active cancer treatment. During follow-up visits, clinicians create a survivorship care plan that is made available to the patient. Survivorship care is provided in close collaboration with patients' primary care clinicians. Jacobs noted that pre- and post-implementation assessments of the program indicate that it has reduced patient wait time, improved clinic capacity, and improved patient satisfaction. She added that patients were satisfied with their care transition from oncologists to APPs and that the program has increased revenue for the health care organization.

Moffitt Cancer Center's Palliative Care Pathways

Diane Portman, chair of the Supportive Care Medicine Department of the Moffitt Cancer Center and professor at the University of South Florida, reported on Moffitt Cancer Center's oncology pathways, which ensure that palliative care is provided to patients at critical junctions during treatment. The pathways were developed internally by consensus among oncologists, palliative care professionals, and individuals with expertise in developing guidelines. At Moffitt, all clinicians on a cancer care team are involved in providing palliative care. An electronic health record alert system prompts clinicians to provide specific specialty level palliative care services in response to patients' health events. Portman noted that embedding palliative care in the pathways program can reduce institutional costs, decrease unnecessary health care usage, and improve patient care (Portman et al., 2018a).

continued

BOX 2 Continued

Sutter Pacific Medical Foundation's Patient Navigation Program
Cynthia Cantril, director of cancer support services and patient navigation at Sutter Pacific Medical Foundation, reported on her institution's patient navigation program. Nurse navigators are assigned to patients at the time of diagnosis and they guide patients through each step in the cancer care process, serving as a central "hub" in the "wheel of cancer care" (see Figure 4). The program endeavors to address patient's psychosocial needs to preemptively provide support. Cantril noted that a key element of the navigation program is its attention to the full continuum of cancer care and its ability to identify and address patients' unique needs at every stage.

Sarah Cannon Research Institute's Nurse Navigation Program
Howard "Skip" Burris, president and chief medical officer of the Sarah Cannon Research Institute, reported on his organization's nurse navigation program. The program has 200 nurse navigators across 14 sites. It focuses on vulnerable populations in the critical period between cancer diagnosis and treatment onset, although navigators continue to engage patients at key transitions through their care. Navigators carry out several tasks, including

- Developing trust with the physicians and patients through multidisciplinary care coordination;
- Assisting in educating patients about their cancer so they can make informed decisions about their care;
- Providing emotional support to the patient, family, and caregivers;
- Improving access and use of Sarah Cannon partners' resources; and
- Advocating for the patient during the development of the treatment plan.

An algorithm is used to analyze patient data and alert clinicians to patients in need of navigation services. Burris reported that the program has reduced institutional costs, improved patient satisfaction and retention, and reduced wait times between diagnosis and treatment.

SOURCES: Burris, Cantril, Jacobs, and Portman presentations, February 11–12, 2019.

(Van Houtven et al., 2019). "We need to quantify these things in order to effect change," Van Houtven said.

Technology Opportunities

A large portion of the workshop was devoted to discussion of new technologies that could support and improve efficiency for patients, caregivers, and clinicians (see Box 3). Topics included the effect of new technologies on cancer care, challenges of implementing new technologies, and strategies to improve EHRs.

The Effect of New Technologies on Cancer Care

Workshop participants discussed ways in which new technologies have changed the delivery of cancer care by improving documentation, patient–clinician communication, health care team functioning, and patient navigation. Technologies that allow for remote patient monitoring and the delivery of telemedicine were discussed in depth. Participants noted that these technologies have begun to change the practice of oncology and will continue to improve care as they are more fully implemented.

Levy pointed out that voice recognition dictation software can relieve some of the tasks of documentation. "We're hoping that eventually the voice recognition is so good that as you are talking to your patient, artificial intelligence programs are placing orders for you to review and verify instead of these asynchronous processes we are currently going through," Levy noted, adding that some groups are currently piloting such systems.

Technology is also enabling easier access of more widespread patient data, Levy pointed out. Much of those data are coming from outside clinicians' own health care systems, but flowing directly into their EHRs. For example, pharmacy data are sent to clinicians about whether their patients are filling their prescriptions, so that clinicians can review and ensure patients are adhering to their medication regimens. Patients can also access their own data via smartphones with apps currently available or being developed.

Dentzer, Levy, Portman, and Takvorian discussed technologies for remote patient monitoring and ways these technologies can be used to improve patient care. Remote patient monitoring allows clinicians to gather information on patients' health and symptoms without requiring in-person clinic visits, reducing patient and caregiver burden. Data collection from remote monitoring technologies can be active (e.g., patients reporting symptoms in a smartphone app) or passive (e.g., data gathered through a wearable device). Dentzer stated that the Veterans Health Administration (VHA) has made significant investments in remote monitoring as part of its "Anywhere to Anywhere" initiative. She noted that more than 150,000 veterans are currently being monitored at

BOX 3
Examples of Technologies to Facilitate Cancer Care

Symptom Care at Home

Kathi Mooney, interim director of the population sciences program and co-leader of the cancer control and population sciences program at the Huntsman Cancer Institute of The University of Utah, reported on Symptom Care at Home (SCH), a program for automated family care support during home-based hospice care. The program provides daily monitoring of the severity of patient symptoms as well as indicators of caregiver well-being. This information is reported by the caregiver via phone. Using algorithms, the program provides tailored family caregiver coaching on strategies to mitigate patient symptoms and improve caregiver well-being. For symptoms that exceed pre-set thresholds, the system sends automated alerts to a hospice nurse for follow-up. Compared with standard hospice care, SCH is associated with reduced symptom severity and enhanced caregiver well-being (Mooney et al., 2017). Mooney reported that patients have reported high satisfaction with the service.

Penny

Samuel Takvorian, chief fellow of the division of hematology and oncology at the Perelman School of Medicine at the University of Pennsylvania, described a program for symptom management and medication adherence—a virtual, artificial intelligence–assisted chat bot called "Penny." Penny engages in real-time conversation with patients via text messaging, offering motivational feedback and advice. Penny provides step-by-step personalized guidance to support oral cancer treatment adherence, including dosing instructions. When patients report symptoms, the system is able to provide self-management advice for low-grade symptoms and it triggers a clinician alert in response to high-grade symptoms. Preliminary testing found high participant satisfaction and improved medication adherence. Use of Penny was also associated with reduced patient call volume.

Project ECHO

Kathleen Schmeler, associate professor of gynecologic oncology and reproductive medicine at The University of Texas MD Anderson Cancer Center, discussed her institution's telementoring program called "Project ECHO" (Extension for Community Healthcare Outcomes). The program was developed to provide specialty care consultations and training to clinicians in low-resource communities. Through telementoring video conferences, specialists can review cases and provide feedback and guidance to community clinicians. Evaluations of the project have shown that community clinicians supported by Project ECHO provide care equal to that provided by academic physicians, and that patients appreciate being able to receive expert medical care without travel. Telementoring builds clinician capacity in low-resource settings, and clinicians who used the program also reported greater self-efficacy and enjoyment in their work (Arora et al., 2011). "The idea of Project ECHO is that it uses technology to spread specialized knowledge—it moves knowledge, not people," Schmeler stressed.

eConsults

Scott Shipman, director of clinical innovations and primary care affairs at the Association of American Medical Colleges, reported on a program called eConsults, which has been implemented at 27 academic medical centers in the United States. He noted that an eConsult is an asynchronous exchange between clinicians that enables a requesting clinician to seek recommendations from a specialist. This allows the requesting clinician to receive and act on medical advice without needing to refer a patient to see a specialist. eConsults can be built into electronic health records or hosted on a Cloud-based platform. Shipman explained that eConsults formalize the consultation process and set clear expectations for an exchange between providers. He noted that the program improves access to specialty care, reduces referrals, and creates a meaningful connection between clinicians, while also reducing the patient burden of establishing care with a new specialist.

Although a 3-year pilot study of CORE's eConsult program found that it saved Medicare approximately $8 million due to reduced specialty visits (Project CORE, 2018), Shipman stressed that "this is not a means of rationing care. If a patient wants to see a specialist, then the referral would happen. But most patients find eConsults a good opportunity for them, given that there is a quick turnaround of 3 days or less for specialist input, and it doesn't require them having to take off of work and travel to a clinic."

RobinCare

Hugh Ma, chief executive officer and founder of RobinCare, Inc., discussed RobinCare, a service for employers and payers that provides a combination of human and virtual navigation and care coordination for patients. Ma noted that many problems patients encounter during cancer treatment are psychosocial and not medical, so he worked to

continued

BOX 3 Continued

create a company that could support patients' needs outside of the clinical team. He stated that there are three principal components of RobinCare:

- 24/7 staffing by a team of cancer experts, including nurse practitioners, financial consultants, mental health counselors, and benefits navigators who are trained in empathy.
- Predictive pathways based on best practices for care that also consider logistical and psychosocial concerns.
- A digital platform that enables online interactions to provide quick responses. Ma noted that this chat feature is an integral part of RobinCare's program.

RobinCare assists patients with functions such as appointments and symptom tracking, and suggests questions to ask during clinical encounters. The system also allows the option of recording patients' conversations with clinicians and providing a lay-friendly summary of the clinician's comments.

SOURCES: Ma, Mooney, Schmeler, Shipman, and Takvorian presentations, February 11, 2019.

home via smartphone, while additional patients are using Fitbits and other wearables to share information with their clinicians. Portman reported that Moffitt has evaluated an app called "Tap Cloud" to collect patient data, which can then be incorporated into EHRs. The app presents patients with a list of symptoms and medication side effects tailored to their disease state and treatment regimen, and allows them to indicate the symptoms and side effects they are experiencing with a few taps of their smartphone. The program also incorporates machine learning tools to personalize the patient experience, identify progression in patients' symptoms, and provide tips on symptoms management.

To interpret data generated by remote monitoring, health care organizations may use algorithms to process patient data and trigger clinical intervention at predetermined thresholds. Portman noted that Moffitt collects and processes data on emotional and physical status to identify patients in need of immediate assistance. Levy described a randomized trial that found a web-based tool for monitoring symptoms at home was able to alert clinicians to disease recurrence and was associated with improved survival compared with standard image-based monitoring; the risk of mortality over a 2-year period was 40 percent lower for patients who used the symptom monitoring tool (Denis et al., 2019). "Most drugs do not have outcomes as good as this," Levy stressed. Takvorian also expressed enthusiasm for the potential of widespread electronic monitoring of patient symptoms, but noted there is an implementation gap as strategies for remote monitoring continue to evolve.

Several workshop participants discussed the use of telemedicine, which allows for remote delivery of clinical services and can improve access to care as well as reduce burdens associated with patient travel. A study of claims data found that telemedicine visits increased by 52 percent annually between 2005 and 2014, and 261 percent annually between 2015 and 2017 (Barnett et al., 2018). Dentzer explained, "A lot of health care requires a laying on of hands, but an awful lot is just about exchanges of information and you can do that virtually so the patient can stay close to home." Telemedicine has become an important tool for expanding access to specialty services in rural areas. Dentzer provided the example of Brattleboro Memorial Hospital, a 61-bed community hospital in southeastern Vermont serving a rural population of 55,000. The hospital maintains a telemedicine linkage to the Dartmouth-Hitchcock Medical Center 71 miles away. Through this connection, Brattleboro Memorial is able to connect with clinicians providing acute specialty care in emergency medicine, intensive care services, neurology, psychiatry, and pharmacy.

Dentzer added that telemedicine can also improve health care access for patients with physical limitations who may have difficulty traveling to an in-person clinic visit. She described a study funded by the Patient-Centered Outcomes Research Institute (PCORI) on virtual care for patients with Parkinson's disease that assessed the effect of integrating telemedicine visits into patients' follow-up care. More than half of the participants preferred the virtual visits to in-person visits, Dentzer noted, adding that these virtual visits relieved transportation and time burdens on patients and their caregivers (Beck et al., 2017). "You can imagine how useful this would be in the context of cancer," Dentzer said.

New technologies have also given patients remote access to palliative care and psychosocial support. Portman noted that Moffitt offers remote palliative care conferencing services to patients for whom distance, cost, or functional status present a burden to travel. Portman noted that patients are satisfied with this form of telepalliative care (Portman et al., 2018b; Worster and Swartz, 2017). Dentzer reported that health care organizations have also reported success with the remote provision of behavioral health care. She noted that the VA is currently conducting a pilot of a telemedicine program to provide remote access to psychotherapy and related services for rural veterans with posttraumatic stress disorder (PTSD). She added that PCORI is also studying the effectiveness of video visits versus in-person visits with a palliative care provider for advanced lung cancer patients.

Dentzer pointed out a number of technologies that are aiding the diagnosis and prognosis of cancer, including systems employing deep learning algorithms that have been shown to outperform pathologists in detecting some types of cancer from biopsies (Liu et al., 2019). She also noted the existence of the crowdsourcing and social networking app Figure1,[6] which enables health care professionals to post and share de-identified medical images and compare opinions and analyses. Dentzer added that crowdsourcing medical knowledge and employing artificial intelligence-aided diagnosis will become much larger components of health care in the future, and will help augment the capacity of individual clinicians to care for patients.

Takvorian added that given the current and future state of apps and other technologies, the smartphone could be considered an important component of the health care team. Patient advocate Joao Salomao agreed and noted that smartphones are used in low-resource areas to send images for expert consultations for cancer diagnosis.

Neal Meropol, vice president of research oncology at Flatiron Health, suggested that novel technologies could also be employed to improve efficiency and reduce patient burden in clinical trials. For example, clinical trial candidates could be identified and monitored through EHRs. "Technology can get us closer to a world where research participation becomes more seamlessly integrated with routine clinical care," Meropol said.

Challenges of Implementing New Technologies

Workshop participants identified challenges of technology implementation and discussed strategies to overcome these challenges. Although new technologies have the potential to mitigate cancer health disparities by improving access to care, there was also concern that they may worsen some disparities if new technologies are not widely available. Leonard Lichtenfeld, acting chief medical and scientific officer at the American Cancer Society, noted that most technologies discussed during the workshop were Internet enabled, and could only be used by patients with access to broadband Internet, which is still unavailable in many rural areas. Dentzer agreed, noting that spotty broadband access is a challenge in ensuring equitable health care.

Dentzer noted that an additional challenge in implementing telehealth more broadly will be laws and regulations that limit home-based care, espe-

---

[6] See https://figure1.com (accessed July 25, 2019).

cially laws concerning state licensure and clinicians' scope of practice. She noted that there are also concerns about privacy and data security because patients' health information is digitally collected and transmitted. Dentzer suggested that full implementation of telehealth will likely require amendments to existing federal and state laws. These potential changes are further explored in the section on Policies to Facilitate the Adoption of New Technologies in Cancer Care.

Several workshop participants identified hesitance of clinicians, patients, and caregivers as a major barrier to technology implementation in cancer care. Dentzer and Takvorian noted that clinicians often are skeptical of new technology. Mooney suggested that some clinicians may see new technologies as a threat to their role in patient care, rather than viewing them as a helpful tool. "We have to involve clinicians very closely [in the development and implementation of a new technology] so they own it," she said. She suggested that educating patients and caregivers about the availability of new technologies for clinical care could help create a demand for their use. "You have to do more than just publish what you have done. You have to create a community that talks about it," Mooney said. Shulman noted that user-friendly technologies are more readily adopted, while Lichtenfeld emphasized that for new technologies to be adopted successfully in health care, they need to either save money or reduce burden for patients, caregivers, or clinicians. Scott Shipman, director of clinical innovations and primary care affairs at the Association of American Medical Colleges, added that new technologies are often not adopted in health care until the problem they are intended to address reaches a point of crisis.

Hugh Ma, CEO and founder of RobinCare, Inc., added that technology often fails in health care because it is viewed as a stand-alone tool, rather than as an all-encompassing integrated service or product. He suggested that it will be important to focus on overall user experience and ease of use, noting that technology needs to serve clinicians and easily facilitate care. Mooney agreed, noting that users will only adopt technologies they find useful. Ma also emphasized the importance of selectively adopting new technologies that provide the highest value, particularly those that have potential to fundamentally improve the delivery of cancer care.

Several participants noted that payers may also resist the implementation of new technologies. Mooney said that although new technologies can save payers money by proactively identifying and addressing health concerns and thus avoiding costly emergency care, reimbursement for these technologies has not been embraced by the traditional fee-for-service payment model. She stated, "Our reimbursement system is missing a huge opportunity to improve the lives of cancer patients because of how it is designed." Shipman agreed, suggesting there should be a shift toward value-based reimbursement or bundled payments that enable clinicians and health care systems more freedom in how they deliver services. But he added that reimbursement for new technologies may be possible in a fee-for-service model if the financial benefits of the new technologies could be clearly demonstrated to a payer. He said that for eConsults, Medicare funded a pilot that allowed the program to gather data to demonstrate its value; at the conclusion of the pilot, CMS agreed to reimburse for the service.

As new technologies are implemented in cancer care, an important consideration is whether applications should be built into EHR systems or created as independent programs. Rosenthal noted that there can be substantial integration costs associated with building new technologies within EHR systems. However, applications that function as independent programs require clinicians to learn and interact with a new interface. Dentzer suggested that new technologies should have common standard elements to facilitate integration in diverse systems. She noted that technology developers and purchasers should predicate all technologies on interoperability, seamless data and information exchange, and data accessibility with appropriate privacy and security safeguards.

Strategies to Improve EHRs

Many participants commented on clinician burden associated with EHR use and proposed strategies to improve EHR design, implementation, and use. Participants frequently commented that EHRs have poor usability, which Sesto defined as "the effectiveness, efficiency, and satisfaction with which specific users can achieve certain tasks in an environment." Sesto added that EHR users are often frustrated by elements of poor design, such as text boxes that are too small to fully display text and requirements for redundant documentation. She noted that poorly designed EHRs are inefficient for their users and may lead to clinical errors. Sesto suggested that many problems with EHR usability could be avoided by testing EHRs with tasks that simulate the real-world complexity of the clinical setting. However, many EHR vendors fail to conduct adequate usability testing (Ratwani et al., 2015). Sesto noted that another common problem in EHR implementation is variability between vendors and across systems. She stated that EHR systems are often tailored by vendors to meet the needs of a particular health care organization, but these customized EHRs may not be evaluated for usability. Sesto noted that the AMA recently partnered with the MedStar Health National Center for Human Factors in Healthcare to provide guidance and information on EHR safety and usability (MedStar Health, 2019).

Sesto also noted that EHRs are not often designed to facilitate effective communication and team-based care. Cox and Nevidjon suggested having a Wiki-like ability to integrate data entered in EHRs by multiple people on a patient's treatment team, in order to avoid the redundancy of patient data entry that often occurs, and to ensure everyone on the team has complete data. This would make care more efficient and address patients' complaints that they are often asked the same questions by different members of a care team, Nevidjon explained.

Sesto noted that current EHRs are typically designed for fee-for-service reimbursement models and will likely need to be redesigned to support the clinical documentation required by value-based reimbursement systems. Paz suggested that vendors could incorporate standardized quality measures into EHRs, including assessments of patient well-being, noting that these quality measures could be used in value-based reimbursements for care. He said this type of reimbursement system would help prioritize care that promotes patients' subjective well-being. Dillon agreed, calling for better measurement of the patient experience during medical care. Scroggins added that it is insufficient to collect data on patient well-being—the information needs to be used to take action. "There's nothing more frustrating than being asked and then realizing that nothing happens," she said.

Sesto stressed that solving the current problems with EHRs cannot be accomplished by a single stakeholder. It will require a multilevel improvement process that includes vendors, clinicians, patients, health care organizations, policy makers, and researchers (Ratwani et al., 2019). Back added, "Our current system is not working. We are at a point where we need some kind of regulation to create real progress because without some real leverage to create that progress, we will continue to have the same glacial pace of change."

Policies to Facilitate the Adoption of New Technologies in Cancer Care

Participants provided several suggestions for policies to facilitate implementation of new technologies in cancer care. Suggestions included a national plan for universal and affordable high-speed broadband, appropriate regulations on patient privacy and data security, regulations and incentives to promote usability in EHRs, and changes to medical licensing and reimbursement structures to enable full implementation of telemedicine.

Noting that many new technologies discussed during the workshop require access to broadband Internet, Dentzer suggested developing a national plan for universal broadband and universal 5G technology. Robert Winn, director of the University of Illinois Cancer Center, agreed, noting that inequalities in access to Internet services have the potential to widen geographic health disparities as Internet services become critical for health care access. Dentzer suggested that every clinician in America should advocate for universal, affordable, high-speed broadband and 5G.

Several workshop participants noted that responsible implementation of new technologies in cancer care will necessitate changes to privacy regulations. Dentzer suggested that the United States should create a national data security and privacy regulation, similar to Europe's General Data Privacy Regulation, particularly to cover the large amounts of electronic health information that are being collected by entities not covered by the Privacy Rule promulgated under the Health Insurance Portability and Accountability Act of 1996.[7]

To encourage human-centered technology design, Dentzer suggested that software developers should adopt voluntary standards for usability. She noted that these standards could be supported by incentives or penalties created by regulatory agencies, including the Food and Drug Administration (FDA). Dentzer also suggested that health care organizations should integrate human factors expertise and human-centered design principles in their strategies and operations. Back suggested that CMS could create new certification requirements for EHRs based on usability. He suggested that ASCO could collaborate with the American Medical Informatics Association (AMIA) to create usability standards to support these new requirements. Sesto reiterated a recommendation made by AMIA to the Department of Health and Human Services[8] that documentation requirements for regulatory and administrative compliance should be separated from clinical documentation. Paz suggested that greater effort should be made across federal agencies and health care systems to standardize quality measures in EHRs and make them easier to report.

Dentzer noted that the implementation of telemedicine is often hindered by licensure restrictions that create geographic limitations on a physician's practice. Some laws restrict the practice of telemedicine within states. To practice across state lines, as telemedicine often requires, physicians must be licensed in both the state in which they practice and the states in which patients are located. Advanced practice registered nurses, by contrast, have created a compact that allows them to have one multistate license that enables practice in all states that have joined the compact. Dentzer suggested that laws and regulations should be modified in every state to enable clinicians to deliver telemedicine consultations across state lines. Acknowledging that state boards may not want to forfeit their ability to control medical licenses, she proposed that the federal government create a national licensure system that states could choose to adopt. "Perhaps over time the state apparatus would wither away as more people saw that national licensure was sufficient," Dentzer said. Dillon

---

[7] For more information on the General Data Privacy Regulation, see https://eugdpr.org (accessed July 19, 2019). For more information on the Privacy Rule, see https://www.hhs.gov/hipaa/for-professionals/privacy/index.html (accessed July 25, 2019).

[8] To read the full comments, see https://www.amia.org/sites/default/files/AMIA-Response-to-ONC-HIT-Burden-Reduction-Strategy.pdf (accessed July 19, 2019).

added that in the absence of new licensing policies, it is important to create professional training to support clinicians in achieving broad licensure. She added that health care professional societies should advocate for a national licensure system.

Dentzer also suggested that payers should develop new payment models to support telemedicine implementation and to encourage substitution of virtual care for in-person care, where appropriate. She suggested that patients could also be incentivized to use virtual technologies that have been shown to improve health outcomes. Payment models are discussed further in the next section.

Policy Opportunities

Workshop participants provided several policy suggestions to restructure payment models, support caregivers, and optimize oncology education, as well as suggesting avenues for future research.

New Payment Models

Several participants noted that existing payment structures are a major barrier to improving oncology care and reducing burden on the careforce. Shulman said that payment is the major driver of change in the U.S. health care system, and finding payment strategies to support innovation is necessary for achieving reproducible and sustainable change. Ronald Kline, medical officer with CMS, noted that payment policies affect the way that health care services are provided, and said some clinical documentation tasks are completed solely for the purpose of meeting insurer requirements.

Within a fee-for-service reimbursement model, health care providers are reimbursed for care based on a medical code associated with each service they provide. Kline, Lichtenfeld, Shulman, and Van Houtven noted that tying payments to the medical coding system limits health care innovation, and often fails to account for or compensate clinicians for important aspects of cancer care, such as the provision of palliative care, clinical encounters with the patient's family, and consultations with other clinicians about a patient's care. "We have to change the way things are reimbursed in order to have this happen, either through performance measures or through alternative payment models," Van Houtven stated.

Mooney suggested that insurers could provide financial incentives for health care systems to implement innovations in care. For example, she suggested that incentives could be provided for the implementation of new technologies that improve patient outcomes. "The right incentives will make more rapid change," she said, noting that previous changes in health care practice have been achieved by addressing payment. Van Houtven also suggested financial incentives that reward team-based metrics rather than individual metrics in oncology care.

Brawley noted that although U.S. health care costs are twice that of its peer countries, many health indicators are worse (OECD, 2011). "We don't get value in our health care," Brawley stated. This cost inefficiency has led to calls to move away from the fee-for-service model and toward value-based reimbursement. Paz said that value-based models promote comprehensive care. He described Aetna's Oncology Medical Home (OMH) program, which incentivizes value-based, comprehensive, patient-centered care (see Box 4). "Rather than focusing on changing the picture, let's look at a new picture. That is ultimately how you wind up solving the problem, because everything we do up until that becomes a halfway solution to try to get there," he said.

BOX 4
Aetna's Oncology Medical Home

Harold Paz, executive vice president and chief medical officer of Aetna, reported on Aetna's Oncology Medical Home (OMH), a value-based care delivery model designed to improve quality and value in oncology care. He noted that OMH focuses on patient experience and encourages health care organizations to innovate to improve patient care. OMHs use a team-based approach that allows every clinician to operate at the top of their license. Compared with traditional oncology care, patients have enhanced access to their care team, including after-hours and weekend contact. For a practice to qualify as an OMH, it must meet size requirements, use Aetna's clinical decision support tools, and have electronic health records. OMHs are also required to use nurse navigators and enhanced triage as well as to report results from patient satisfaction surveys.

Aetna rewards practices that commit to developing an OMH by allowing them to share in cost savings. Individual physicians are also rewarded for improved health outcomes, including reduced inpatient hospital stays and reduced emergency room visits for adverse events associated with chemotherapy.

Aetna currently has 22 OMHs across 18 states that include 750 oncologists. Paz said this growth reflects Aetna's commitment to facilitate the delivery of high-quality, patient-centered oncology while moving toward value-based care.

SOURCE: Paz presentation, February 12, 2019.

Workshop participants identified many advantages of value-based payment models. Cox suggested that value-based payment would shift medical practice toward patient-centric care and away from billing-centric care. He noted that many effective oncology practices cannot be reimbursed within a fee-for-service model and are therefore viewed as a revenue loss. A value-based system would support these services because they improve patient outcomes while reducing overall cost and complexity of care. However, Shulman noted that value-based reimbursement may be a better fit for discrete episodes of health care (e.g., a hip replacement) that have a clear beginning and end than for long-term or chronic diseases such as cancer. Kline agreed, noting that both the cost of cancer drugs and standard of care change rapidly in oncology. He said the Oncology Care Model[9] considers the increasing costs of drugs and makes annual adjustments to its reimbursements. "Oncology is hard because there isn't a defined starting and stopping point, so that is why we created 6-month episodes of care. Those episodes can repeat as long as you continue treating a patient," Kline said.

Dillon suggested that community cancer advocates and organizations can be partners in raising patient voices for state or federal action. "We can bring that voice forward to effect change in reimbursement and make sure the patient's perspective is always included when we are talking about following clinical pathways and trying to save dollars," Dillon said.

Support for Caregivers

Van Houtven suggested that one strategy to develop and sustain an effective and resilient oncology careforce is to create policies that provide support for patients' caregivers (NASEM, 2016). She called for an expansion of guaranteed leave policies to allow caregivers to take time off from work while retaining their employment. However, she noted that unpaid leave is often insufficient, particularly for low-income families who are more vulnerable to lost income (Wolff et al., 2019). To further reduce negative consequences for caregivers, Van Houtven called for programs to provide caregivers with financial support, for example, paid family leave and caregiving tax credits. She noted that although some state Medicaid programs and the VHA allow payments for caregivers, her research found that only about 3 percent of caregivers receive any kind of financial support. Van Houtven also suggested implementing lifetime cost caps on insurance to reduce financial burden for patients and caregiver spouses. She said,

---

[9] For more information on the CMS Oncology Care Model, see https://innovation.cms.gov/initiatives/oncology-care (accessed September 4, 2019).

People who are doing well and are wealthier are the ones who are able to access and pay for services, so we have to identify policy levers to target scarce resources to those who are least resilient in the fact of cancer diagnosis, especially those family members and friends who pitch in.

Education

Several workshop participants identified opportunities to leverage education and training to provide high-quality oncology care that meets the needs of the growing population of cancer survivors. One set of suggestions focused on changes to professional education to extend workforce capacity, reduce burnout, and maximize quality of care. Participants also discussed strategies to build the future cancer workforce through primary and secondary education.

Professional education   Shulman noted that medical school and nursing school curricula often focus on the basic biology and pathogenesis of disease and devote little attention to practice-related issues such as how to interact with other professionals on a team. Van Houtven agreed, suggesting that education should also address best practices for communication among specialties. She noted, "We are good at breaking things up and assigning different tasks to different experts, but we're not so good at reintegrating. What relay team would forget to train their people in handing off the baton?" Portman and Back suggested there should be more clinician training in patient communication, noting that strong communication skills can enhance clinician well-being. Jill Lowery, acting chief of ethics policy at the National Center for Ethics in Health Care at the VHA, described the program she leads called the Life-Sustaining Treatment Decisions Initiative, which builds clinicians' skills in communicating with seriously ill patients (see Box 5). In addition to interprofessional and patient communication skills, Portman noted the importance of including palliative care training for all cancer clinicians; she suggested including palliative care in continuing education and boarding curricula for all new hires. Van Houtven proposed that oncology organizations and professional societies, such as ASCO and ONS, could serve as partners in developing new clinical curricula.

Hyde suggested that an important strategy for increasing oncology care capacity is training APPs to allow them to practice more autonomously. He noted that there is no formal post-graduate accreditation system for oncology APPs, and suggested that this training could take the form of a fellowship, residency, or other structured post-graduate program. He added that financial incentives could also be used to encourage health care organizations to maximize APPs' autonomy, and suggested formal trainings for oncology clinicians

BOX 5
The Life-Sustaining Treatment Decisions Initiative
of the Veterans Health Administration

Jill Lowery, acting chief of ethics policy at the National Center for Ethics in Health Care at the Department of Veterans Affairs, reported on the Veterans Health Administration's (VHA's) Life-Sustaining Treatment Decisions Initiative. This program is designed to standardize practices around eliciting, documenting, and honoring patients' goals of care and preferences about life-sustaining treatments.

To assist clinicians in delivering serious news, conducting goals of care conversations, and making shared decisions with patients about life-sustaining treatments, the VHA developed a series of communication skills training modules. The training programs are designed to improve communication around serious illness, and include didactics as well as interactive practice that is critical for skill building.

The Delivering Serious News/Goals of Care Conversation training program for physicians, nurse practitioners, and physician assistants has five interactive modules, each 45 to 50 minutes long, which may be delivered together or over a series of short sessions. The training program for nurses, social workers, psychologists, and chaplains is customized to their scope of practice, and consists of three modules. One module in this program helps teams develop systematic approaches to proactively identify high-risk patients, prepare patients and their families for these conversations, and ensure accurate and comprehensive documentation. Clinicians have given the trainings high ratings.

Lowery reported that during the first 2 years of the program, more than 120,000 patients have had goals of care conversations and developed life-sustaining treatment plans. In addition, more than 750 clinicians nationwide have completed a training on how to teach the training program at their home institutions. All of the materials from the program are publicly available and downloadable.[a]

---

[a] For more information on the VA training programs, see https://www.ethics.va.gov/goalsofcaretraining/Practitioner.asp (accessed September 4, 2019).
SOURCE: Lowery presentation, February 11, 2019.

on how to optimize the role of PAs and NPs in oncology practice. Nevidjon suggested focusing on oncology training for nurses as well. She noted that the ONS has developed and is currently evaluating resources for pre-licensure oncology training programs. ONS has also developed a post-master's degree course on oncology nursing for non-oncology NPs.

Carlson suggested that health care organizations should establish formal mentoring programs to support early-career oncology clinicians, defining mentorship as a developmental, empowering, and nurturing relationship extending over time in which there is mutual sharing, learning, and growth. Carlson noted that mentoring is likely to be reciprocal—both mentor and mentee share knowledge, insight, and skills (Fielden et al., 2009). He reported that in academic medicine, mentees are more likely to be successful and productive, and have higher retention rates and career satisfaction (Cho et al., 2011).

Primary and secondary education   Several participants noted that an additional strategy to grow the future oncology workforce is to generate interest in the cancer care professions early in the educational pipeline. Shulman observed that fewer medical students and early career clinicians are choosing to specialize in oncology. Winn noted that it could be fruitful to encourage high school– and middle school–aged students to consider cancer care professions. Shulman said the University of Pennsylvania has a program to teach high school students about cancer medicine, with the hope of building interest for a future career. He said the program has been well received, but cautioned that merely increasing the number of cancer care clinicians may be insufficient to address current shortcomings in cancer care.

Brawley also advocated for including lessons in cancer prevention for children, even as early as preschool. He suggested implementing educational programs to encourage healthy behaviors such as exercise and healthy diet, which have the potential to reduce cancer risk and thus reduce the number of future cancer patients. Nevidjon suggested partnering with teachers, counselors, and school nurses to deliver this curriculum. She added that cancer prevention education in the schools might also encourage more students to choose nursing as a profession, noting that the National Student Nurses Association already partners with school systems to encourage students to pursue nursing.

Patients and the public also need to be more educated about palliative care, Scroggins noted. She said many patients have the misconception that palliative care is only appropriate at the end of life. Scroggins also suggested educating patients in health literacy, which she described as "the language of medicine, the language of cancer, understanding the things we need to know to gain access and be able to ask the right kinds of questions."

Future Research

Workshop participants made several suggestions regarding avenues for future research, including research on the effects of caregiving; care delivery and care teams; multimodal care; implementation science; and the effects of new treatments, programs, and technologies.

Van Houtven noted that although most people in the oncology community believe high-quality caregiving improves patient outcomes, the association has not been directly studied. She suggested that empirical evidence of the benefits of caregiving would facilitate implementation of programs that provide caregivers with financial and psychosocial support. Cox suggested additional research on how cancer care is delivered, including research on the role of team care. Bruinooge agreed and added that there is a lack of research on patient outcomes from multimodality cancer treatments, noting that studies on cancer drugs, surgery, and radiation treatment are often siloed, so there is little research showing how these modalities could most optimally be combined and sequenced.

Several workshop participants discussed the need for further research demonstrating the effects of new oncology care programs and technologies. "Tools are wonderful and we often think adoption of those tools is good and correct. But how do we actually know that the tools themselves are having the impact we hoped they would have, or whether they are having a different impact than what we were expecting?" Levy asked. Other participants called for research to demonstrate the patient care and cost savings benefits associated with programs such as patient navigation, palliative care, and survivorship care. Shulman noted that to support the implementation of these programs, it will be important to prove they reduce cost and improve quality.

Van Houtven noted the importance of studying implementation science, and suggested that organizations such as ASCO, the National Institutes of Health, the National Cancer Institute, PCORI, and CMS are valuable partners for this endeavor. Sarah Birken, assistant professor at the University of North Carolina at Chapel Hill, agreed, noting that many promising technologies are never implemented or are implemented poorly. "There is a science of implementation and it needs to be harnessed if we are going to make good on all of the innovation you are talking about," she said.

WRAP-UP

Shulman provided the workshop wrap-up, in which he summarized the discussion and suggested next steps for developing and sustaining the oncology careforce. He noted that delivering high-quality patient care is the goal for all oncology clinicians, but oncology is challenged by the growing number of patients and limited number of clinicians. Shulman suggested that the oncology field needs to identify efficient and sustainable models of care to address this pending careforce shortage. One strategy for improving efficiency is to promote interdisciplinary teamwork among clinicians, patient navigators, pharmacists, psychosocial professionals, caregivers, and patients. Shulman noted that workshop participants had offered several promising ideas for reorganizing oncology care, but additional effort is needed to identify the best strategies for implementation. Many workshop participants noted that the transition from fee-for-service to value-based reimbursement models will be pivotal in the adoption of new programs and technologies. Shulman added that the current reimbursement system is a burden to both payers and clinicians and serves as an impediment to care improvement.

Shulman also suggested that improving patient care will require redesigning EHRs to reduce clinician burden, noting that important clinical data are often difficult to access. He stated that many other technologies discussed at the workshop also have the potential to improve support for patients, clinicians, and caregivers as well to improve efficiency of care. Shulman stressed that technology needs to be designed and implemented in partnership with the oncology careforce.

Shulman ended his remarks by quoting Winston Churchill, who said, "Difficulties mastered are opportunities won." He suggested that participants should work to turn the difficulties discussed at the workshop into opportunities to support the oncology careforce and optimize the delivery of high-quality oncology care.

REFERENCES

AACR (American Association for Cancer Research). 2018. *AACR cancer progress report.* https://www.cancerprogressreport.org/Pages/default.aspx (accessed May 16, 2019).

AAPA (American Academy of PAs) Research Department. 2018. *Are PAs burned out?* https://www.aapa.org/news-central/2018/05/pas-report-low-burnout (accessed May 31, 2019).

ACCC (Association of Community Cancer Centers). 2017. *2017 trending now in cancer care survey.* https://www.accc-cancer.org/home/learn/publications/Trends/2017-trending-now-in-cancer-care-survey (accessed July 19, 2019).

ACS (American Cancer Society). 2016. *Cancer treatment & survivorship facts & figures 2016–2017.* https://www.cancer.org/content/dam/cancer-org/research/cancer-facts-and-statistics/cancer-treatment-and-survivorship-facts-and-figures/cancer-treatment-and-survivorship-facts-and-figures-2016-2017.pdf (accessed July 24, 2019).

AMA (American Medical Association). 2018. *2018 AMA Prior Authorization (PA) physician survey.* https://www.ama-assn.org/system/files/2019-02/prior-auth-2018.pdf (accessed July 18, 2019).

Arora, S., K. Thornton, G. Murata, P. Deming, S. Kalishman, D. Dion, B. Parish, T. Burke, W. Pak, J. Dunkelberg, M. Kistin, J. Brown, S. Jenkusky, M. Komaromy, and C. Qualls. 2011. Outcomes of treatment for hepatitis C virus infection by primary care providers. *New England Journal of Medicine* 364(23):2199–2207.

ASCO (American Society of Clinical Oncology), Harris Poll on behalf of ASCO. 2018. *National Cancer Opinion Survey.* Rochester, NY: Harris Insights & Analytics LLC, A Stagwell Company.

Ashkenas, R. N., and B. Manville. 2018. *Harvard Business Review Leader's Handbook: Make an impact, inspire your organization, and get to the next level.* Brighton, MA: Harvard Business Review Press.

Back, A. L., K. E. Steinhauser, A. H. Kamal, and V. A. Jackson. 2016. Building resilience for palliative care clinicians: An approach to burnout prevention based on individual skills and workplace factors. *Journal of Pain and Symptom Management* 52(2):284–291.

Ballas, L. K., E. B. Elkin, D. Schrag, B. D. Minsky, and P. B. Bach. 2006. Radiation therapy facilities in the United States. *International Journal of Radiation Oncology Biology Physics* 66(4):1204–1211.

Banker, R. D., J. M. Field, R. G. Schroeder, and K. K. Sintia. 1996. Impact of work teams on manufacturing performance: A longitudinal field study. *The Academy of Management Journal* 39(4):867–890.

Barnett, M. L., K. N. Ray, J. Souza, and A. Mehrotra. 2018. Trends in telemedicine use in a large commercially insured population, 2005–2017. *JAMA* 320(20):2147–2149.

Beck, C. A., D. B. Beran, K. M. Biglan, C. M. Boyd, E. R. Dorsey, P. N. Schmidt, R. Simone, A. W. Willis, N. B. Galifianakis, M. Katz, C. M. Tanner, K. Dodenhoff, J. Aldred, J. Carter, A. Fraser, J. Jimenez-Shahed, C. Hunter, M. Spindler, S. Reichwein, Z. Mari, B. Dunlop, J. C. Morgan, D. McLane, P. Hickey, L. Gauger, I. H. Richard, N. I. Mejia, G. Bwala, M. Nance, L. C. Shih, C. Singer, S. Vargas-Parra, C. Zadikoff, N. Okon, A. Feigin, J. Ayan, C. Vaughan, R. Pahwa, R. Dhall, A. Hassan, S. DeMello, S. S. Riggare, P. Wicks, M. A. Achey, M. J. Elson, S. Goldenthal, H. T. Keenan, R. Korn, H. Schwarz, S. Sharma, E. A. Stevenson, and W. Zhu. 2017. National randomized controlled trial of virtual house calls for Parkinson disease. *Neurology* 89(11):1152–1161.

Bruinooge, S. S., T. A. Pickard, W. Vogel, A. Hanley, C. Schenkel, E. Garrett-Mayer, E. Tetzlaff, M. Rosenzweig, H. Hylton, S. N. Westin, N. Smith, C. Lynch, M. P. Kosty, and S. F. Williams. 2018. Understanding the Role of Advanced Practice Providers in Oncology in the United States. *Journal of Oncology Practice* 14(9):e518–e532.

Burwell, S. M. 2015. Setting value-based payment goals—HHS efforts to improve US health care. *New England Journal of Medicine* 372(10):897–899.

Cacioppo, J. T., and S. Cacioppo. 2014. Older adults reporting social isolation or loneliness show poorer cognitive function 4 years later. *Evidence-Based Nursing* 17(2):59–60.

Casalino, L. P., D. Gans, R. Weber, M. Cea, A. Tuchovsky, T. F. Bishop, Y. Miranda, B. A. Frankel, K. B. Ziehler, M. M. Wong, and T. B. Evenson. 2016. U.S. physician practices spend more than $15.4 billion annually to report quality measures. *Health Affairs* 35(3):401–406.

Castka, P., C. F. Bamber, F. M. Sharp, and P. Belohoubek. 2001. Factors affecting successful implementation of high performance teams. *Team Performance Management: An International Journal* 7:123–134.

CDC (Centers for Disease Control and Prevention). 2018. National Center for Chronic Disease Prevention and Health Promotion, Division of Population Health. *Chronic Disease Indicators (CDI) data.* https://nccd.cdc.gov/cdi (accessed July 2, 2019).

Cho, C. S., R. A. Ramanan, and M. D. Feldman. 2011. Defining the ideal qualities of mentorship: A qualitative analysis of the characteristics of outstanding mentors. *The American Journal of Medicine* 124(5):453–458.

Colditz, G. A., K. Y. Wolin, and S. Gehlert. 2012. Applying what we know to accelerate cancer prevention. *Science Translational Medicine* 4(127):1–9.

de Moor, J. S., E. C. Dowling, D. U. Ekwueme, G. P. Guy, Jr., J. Rodriguez, K. S. Virgo, X. Han, E. E. Kent, C. Li, K. Litzelman, T. S. McNeel, B. Liu, and K. R. Yabroff. 2017. Employment implications of informal cancer caregiving. *Journal of Cancer Survivorship: Research and Practice* 11(1):48–57.

Denis, F., E. Basch, A.-L. Septans, J. Bennouna, T. Urban, A. C. Dueck, and C. Letellier. 2019. Two-year survival comparing web-based symptom monitoring vs routine surveillance following treatment for lung cancer effects on survival of web-based symptom monitoring vs routine surveillance after lung cancer treatment letters. *JAMA* 321(3):306–307.

Downing, N. L., D. W. Bates, and C. A. Longhurst. 2018. Physician burnout in the EHR era: Are we ignoring the real cause? *Annals of Internal Medicine* 169(1):50–51.

Edmondson, A. 1999. Psychological safety and learning behavior in work teams. *Administrative Science Quarterly* 44(2):350–383.

Erikson, C., E. Salsberg, G. Forte, S. Bruinooge, and M. Goldstein. 2007. Future supply and demand for oncologists: Challenges to assuring access to oncology services. *Journal of Oncology Practice* 3(2):79–86.

Federman, A. D., T. Soones, L. V. DeCherrie, B. Leff, and A. L. Siu. 2018. Association of a bundled hospital-at-home and 30-day postacute transitional care program with clinical outcomes and patient experiences. *JAMA Internal Medicine* 178(8):1033–1040.

Ferrell, B. R., M. L. Twaddle, A. Melnick, and D. E. Meier. 2018. National consensus project clinical practice guidelines for quality palliative care guidelines, 4th edition. *Journal of Palliative Medicine* 21(12):1684–1689.

Fielden, S. L., M. J. Davidson, and V. J. Sutherland. 2009. Innovations in coaching and mentoring: Implications for nurse leadership development. *Health Services Management Research* 22(2):92–99.

Greer, J. A., N. Amoyal, L. Nisotel, J. N. Fishbein, J. MacDonald, J. Stagl, I. Lennes, J. S. Temel, S. A. Safren, and W. F. Pirl. 2016. A systematic review of adherence to oral antineoplastic therapies. *The Oncologist* 21(3):354–376.

HHS (Department of Health and Human Services), Health Resources and Services Administration, and National Center for Health Workforce Analysis. 2017. *National and regional supply and demand projections of the nursing workforce: 2014–2020.* Rockville, MD: HHS, Health Resources and Services Administration, and the National Center for Health Workforce Analysis.

IOM (Institute of Medicine). 2006. *From cancer patient to cancer survivor: Lost in transition.* Washington, DC: The National Academies Press.

IOM. 2009. *Ensuring quality cancer care through the oncology workforce: Sustaining care in the 21st century: Workshop summary.* Washington, DC: The National Academies Press.

IOM. 2013a. *Delivering high-quality cancer care: Charting a new course for a system in crisis.* Washington, DC: The National Academies Press.

IOM. 2013b. *Reducing tobacco-related cancer incidence and mortality: Workshop summary.* Washington, DC: The National Academies Press.

IOM. 2015. *Vital signs: Core metrics for health and health care progress.* Washington, DC: The National Academies Press.

Kamal, K. M., J. R. Covvey, A. Dashputre, S. Ghosh, S. Shah, M. Bhosle, and C. Zacker. 2017. A systematic review of the effect of cancer treatment on work productivity of patients and caregivers. *Journal of Managed Care & Specialty Pharmacy* 23(2):136–162.

Kirkwood, M. K., A. Hanley, S. S. Bruinooge, E. Garrett-Mayer, L. A. Levit, C. Schenkel, J. E. Seid, B. N. Polite, and R. L. Schilsky. 2018. The state of oncology practice in America, 2018: Results of the ASCO practice census survey. *Journal of Oncology Practice* 14(7):e412–e420.

Krasner, M. S., R. M. Epstein, H. Beckman, A. L. Suchman, B. Chapman, C. J. Mooney, and T. E. Quill. 2009. Association of an educational program in mindful communication with burnout, empathy, and attitudes among primary care physicians. *JAMA* 302(12):1284–1293.

Lehn, J. M., R. D. Gerkin, S. C. Kisiel, L. O'Neill, and S. T. Pinderhughes. 2018. Pharmacists providing palliative care services: Demonstrating a positive return on investment. *Journal of Palliative Medicine* 22(6):644–648.

Liu, Y., T. Kohlberger, M. Norouzi, G. E. Dahl, J. L. Smith, A. Mohtashamian, N. Olson, L. H. Peng, J. D. Hipp, and M. C. Stumpe. 2019. Artificial intelligence-based breast cancer nodal metastasis detection: Insights into the black box for pathologists. *Archives of Pathology & Laboratory Medicine* 143(7):859–868.

Maslach, C., and S. E. Jackson. 1981. The measurement of experienced burnout. *Journal of Organizational Behavior* 2(2):99–113.

McDonnell, S. 2017. *America's nurses are aging.* https://alliedstaffingnetwork.com/americas-nurses-are-aging (accessed May 16, 2019).

McFarland, D. C., J. Holland, and R. F. Holcombe. 2015. Inpatient hematology–oncology rotation is associated with a decreased interest in pursuing an oncology career among internal medicine residents. *Journal of Oncology Practice* 11(4):289–295.

MedStar Health. 2019. *Electronic health record (EHR) safety and usability.* https://ehrseewhatwemean.org (accessed July 19, 2019).

Mollica, M. A., K. Litzelman, J. H. Rowland, and E. E. Kent. 2017. The role of medical/nursing skills training in caregiver confidence and burden: A CanCORS study. *Cancer* 123(22):4481–4487.

Mooney, K. H., S. L. Beck, B. Wong, W. Dunson, D. Wujcik, M. Whisenant, and G. Donaldson. 2017. Automated home monitoring and management of patient-reported symptoms during chemotherapy: Results of the symptom care at home RCT. *Cancer Medicine* 6(3):537–546.

NASEM (National Academies of Sciences, Engineering, and Medicine). 2015. *Improving diagnosis in health care.* Washington, DC: The National Academies Press.

NASEM. 2016. *Families caring for an aging America.* Washington, DC: The National Academies Press.

NASEM. 2018a. *Improving cancer diagnosis and care: Patient access to oncologic imaging and pathology expertise and technologies: Proceedings of a workshop.* Washington, DC: The National Academies Press.

NASEM. 2018b. *Incorporating weight management and physical activity throughout the cancer care continuum: Proceedings of a workshop.* Washington, DC: The National Academies Press.

National Alliance for Caregiving and the AARP Public Policy Institute. 2015. *Caregiving in the U.S.: 2015 Report.* https://www.caregiving.org/Caregiving2015 (accessed September 4, 2019).

NCP (National Consensus Project for Quality Palliative Care). 2018. *Clinical practice guidelines for quality palliative care, 4th edition.* Richmond, VA: National Coalition for Hospice and Palliative Care. https://www.nationalcoalitionhpc.org/ncp (accessed July 22, 2019).

OECD (Organisation for Economic Co-operation and Development). 2011. *Health at a glance 2011.* https://doi.org/10.1787/health_glance-2011-en (accessed September 4, 2019).

Ommaya, A. K., P. F. Cipriano, D. B. Hoyt, K. A. Horvath, P. Tang, H. L. Paz, M. S. DeFrancesco, S. T. Hingle, S. Butler, and C. A. Sinsky. 2018. Care-centered clinical documentation in the digital environment: Solutions to alleviate burnout. *NAM Perspectives.* Discussion Paper, National Academy of Medicine, Washington, DC.

Passel, J., and D. Cohn. 2008. *US population projections: 2005–2050.* Washington, DC: Pew Hispanic Center.

Porath, C. 2016. *The hidden toll of workplace incivility.* https://www.mckinsey.com/business-functions/organization/our-insights/the-hidden-toll-of-workplace-incivility (accessed July 19, 2019).

Porath, C., and C. Pearson. 2013. The price of incivility. *Harvard Business Review* 91(1–2):114–121, 146.

Portman, D., S. Siderow, and K. de Lisle. 2018a. *Standardizing palliative care and oncology integration using assessments and care pathways: Moffitt Cancer Center's approach.* Accountable Care Learning Collaborative. https://www.accountablecarelc.org/sites/default/files/ACLC_CSB_Moffitt_Final_0.pdf (accessed July 2, 2019).

Portman, D., S. Thirlwell, and K. A. Donovan. 2018b. Completing the bucket list: Leveraging telemedicine in oncologic palliative care to support legacy-making and dignity. *Journal of Pain and Symptom Management* 55(6):e1–e2.

President's Cancer Panel. 2018. Promoting value, affordability, and innovation in cancer drug treatment. A report to the President of the United States. https://prescancerpanel.cancer.gov/report/drugvalue (accessed August 5, 2019).

Project CORE (Coordinating Optimal Referral Experiences). 2018 (unpublished). Final Awardee Report to Center for Medicare & Medicaid Innovation.

Ratwani, R. M., N. C. Benda, A. Z. Hettinger, and R. J. Fairbanks. 2015. Electronic health record vendor adherence to usability certification requirements and testing standards. *JAMA* 314(10):1070–1071.

Ratwani, R. M., J. Reider, and H. Singh. 2019. A decade of health information technology usability challenges and the path forward. *JAMA* 321(8):743–744.

Reblin, M., B. R. W. Baucom, M. F. Clayton, R. Utz, M. Caserta, D. Lund, K. Mooney, and L. Ellington. 2019. Communication of emotion in home hospice cancer care: Implications for spouse caregiver depression into bereavement. *Journal of the Psychological, Social, and Behavioral Dimensions of Cancer* 28(5):1102–1109.

Rosland, A. M., and J. D. Piette. 2010. Emerging models for mobilizing family support for chronic disease management: A structured review. *Chronic Illness* 6(1):7–21.

Shanafelt, T. D., O. Hasan, L. N. Dyrbye, C. Sinsky, D. Satele, J. Sloan, and C. P. West. 2015. Changes in burnout and satisfaction with work–life balance in physicians and the general U.S. working population between 2011 and 2014. *Mayo Clinic Proceedings* 90(12):1600–1613.

Shanafelt, T. D., L. N. Dyrbye, C. Sinsky, O. Hasan, D. Satele, J. Sloan, and C. P. West. 2016. Relationship between clerical burden and characteristics of the electronic environment with physician burnout and professional satisfaction. *Mayo Clinic Proceedings* 91(7):836–848.

Shulman, L. N., L. A. Jacobs, S. Greenfield, B. Jones, M. S. McCabe, K. Syrjala, L. Diller, C. L. Shapiro, A. C. Marcus, M. Campbell, S. Santacroce, M. Kagawa-Singer, and P. A. Ganz. 2009. Cancer care and cancer survivorship care in the United States: Will we be able to care for these patients in the future? *Journal of Oncology Practice* 5(3):119–123.

Siegel, R. L., K. D. Miller, and A. Jemal. 2018. Cancer statistics, 2018. *CA: A Cancer Journal for Clinicians* 68(1):7–30.

Silliman, R., S. Bhatti, A. Khan, K. A. Dukes, and L. M. Sullivan. 1996. The care of older persons with diabetes mellitus: Families and primary care physicians. *Journal of the American Geriatrics Society* 44(11):1314–1321.

Smiley, R. A., P. Lauer, C. Bienemy, J. G. Berg, E. Shireman, K. A. Reneau, and M. Alexander. 2018. The 2017 national nursing workforce survey. *Journal of Nursing Regulation* 9(3):S1–S88.

Van Houtven, C. H., S. D. Ramsey, M. C. Hornbrook, A. A. Atienza, and M. van Ryn. 2010. Economic burden for informal caregivers of lung and colorectal cancer patients. *Oncologist* 15(8):883–893.

Van Houtven, C. H., S. N. Hastings, and G. Colón-Emeric. 2019. A path to high-quality team-based care for people with serious illness. *Health Affairs* 38(6):934–940.

van Ryn, M., S. Sanders, K. Kahn, C. van Houtven, J. M. Griffin, M. Martin, A. A. Atienza, S. Phelan, D. Finstad, and J. Rowland. 2011. Objective burden, resources, and other stressors among informal cancer caregivers: A hidden quality issue? *Psychooncology* 20(1):44–52.

Waller, A., A. Girgis, C. Johnson, C. Lecathelinais, D. Sibbritt, D. Forstner, W. Liauw, and D. C. Currow. 2012. Improving outcomes for people with progressive cancer: Interrupted time series trial of a needs assessment intervention. *Journal of Pain and Symptom Management* 43(3):569–581.

Weir, H. K., T. D. Thompson, A. Soman, B. Moller, and S. Leadbetter. 2015a. The past, present, and future of cancer incidence in the United States: 1975 through 2020. *Cancer* 121(11):1827–1837.

Weir, H. K., T. D. Thompson, A. Soman, B. Moller, S. Leadbetter, and M. C. White. 2015b. Meeting the Healthy People 2020 objectives to reduce cancer mortality. *Preventing Chronic Disease* 12:E104.

Wolff, J. L., B. C. Spillman, V. A. Freedman, and J. D. Kasper. 2016. A national profile of family and unpaid caregivers who assist older adults with health care activities. *JAMA Internal Medicine* 176(3):372–379.

Wolff, J. L., E. F. Drabo, and C. H. Van Houtven. 2019. Beyond parental leave: Paid family leave for an aging America. *Journal of the American Geriatrics Society* 67(7):1322–1324.

Worster, B., and K. Swartz. 2017. Telemedicine and palliative care: An increasing role in supportive oncology. *Current Oncology Reports* 19(6):37.

Yang, W., J. H. Williams, P. F. Hogan, S. S. Bruinooge, G. I. Rodriguez, M. P. Kosty, D. F. Bajorin, A. Hanley, A. Muchow, N. McMillan, and M. Goldstein. 2014. Projected supply of and demand for oncologists and radiation oncologists through 2025: An aging, better-insured population will result in shortage. *Journal of Oncology Practice* 10(1):39–45.

Zerillo, J. A., B. A. Goldenberg, R. R. Kotecha, A. K. Tewari, J. O. Jacobson, and M. K. Krzyzanowska. 2018. Interventions to improve oral chemotherapy safety and quality: A systematic review. *JAMA Oncology* 4(1):105–117.

Appendix A

Statement of Task

An ad hoc committee will plan and host a 1.5-day public workshop that will examine the impact of evolving trends in cancer incidence and care on the oncology careforce and consider opportunities to enhance patient care through improved development and support of the careforce. The workshop will feature invited presentations and panel discussions on topics that may include

- Factors in the oncology care setting that contribute to inefficiencies, clinician burnout, and reduced quality of care (e.g., electronic health records, documentation and other regulatory requirements, and pre-authorizations), as well as potential systems interventions to address these issues.
- Approaches to stratify and optimize care across the cancer care continuum (e.g., for new versus returning patients on active treatment versus survivorship care).
- The impact of new payment models, such as the Centers for Medicare & Medicaid Services' Oncology Care Model.
- Approaches to improve the recruitment, training, mentorship, and retention of oncology care professionals.
- Approaches to enhance cancer care competencies across the spectrum of non-oncology care providers, from physicians and advanced practice nurses to family caregivers.
- Opportunities for collaboration and information sharing among health care providers (e.g., physicians, nurses, home health care workers, and family caregivers) and across clinical specialties (e.g., oncology, primary

care, cardiology, endocrinology) to identify best practices for careforce coordination and utilization.

The committee will develop the agenda for the workshop sessions, select and invite speakers and discussants, and moderate the discussions. A proceedings of the presentations and discussions at the workshop will be prepared by a designated rapporteur in accordance with institutional guidelines.

Appendix B

Workshop Agenda

February 11, 2019

7:30 am   **Registration and Breakfast**

8:00 am   **Welcome from the National Cancer Policy Forum and Workshop Overview**
Lisa Kennedy Sheldon, Oncology Nursing Society
Lawrence Shulman, University of Pennsylvania
Planning Committee Co-Chairs

8:10 am   **Session 1: Cancer Demographic and Careforce Trends and Implications for the Future of Cancer Care**
Moderator: Randall Oyer, Penn Medicine Lancaster General Health

- **Current and projected trends in cancer incidence, prevalence, and patient care needs**
     Otis Brawley, Johns Hopkins University

- **Current and projected trends of the cancer careforce**
     Suanna Steeby Bruinooge, American Society of Clinical Oncology
     Brenda Nevidjon, Oncology Nursing Society

- **Optimizing the contribution of family caregivers in the oncology careforce**
  Courtney Harold Van Houtven, Duke University and Department of Veterans Affairs

- **The changing nature of cancer care, its impact on the careforce, and envisioning the optimal cancer careforce of the future**
  Lawrence Shulman, University of Pennsylvania

Panel Discussion

10:15 am   **Break**

10:30 am   **Session 2: Improving Cancer Care by Addressing Work System Factors That Contribute to Clinician Burnout and Poor-Quality Care**
Moderator: Lawrence Shulman, University of Pennsylvania

- **Addressing health care practice and organizational factors in cancer care**
  Robert Carlson, National Comprehensive Cancer Network

- **Improving clinician well-being and resilience and addressing recruitment and retention challenges**
  Anthony L. Back, University of Washington and Fred Hutchinson Cancer Research Center

- **Preparing the workforce for collaborative, interprofessional practice and optimizing the way members of the cancer careforce spend their time**
  John Cox, University of Texas Southwestern Medical Center

- **Reducing administrative burdens and documentation requirements**
  Harold Paz, Aetna

- **Improving the design and usability of electronic health records and clinical decision support for clinicians, patients, and families**
  Mary Sesto, University of Wisconsin–Madison

Panel Discussion

12:35 pm   Lunch

1:15 pm   **Session 3: Care Delivery Models to Effectively Leverage
the Cancer Careforce and Optimize Care**
Moderator: Lori Hoffman Hōgg, Department of Veterans
Affairs

- **Advanced practice provider dedicated survivorship/
follow-up care clinics**
Linda Jacobs, University of Pennsylvania

- **Innovations in palliative care to support an effective
and resilient oncology careforce**
Diane Portman, Moffitt Cancer Center

- **Redesigning care by leveraging patient navigation**
Cynthia Cantril, Sutter Pacific Medical Foundation

Panel Discussion
Includes speakers and
Mary Jackson Scroggins, Pinkie Hugs, LLC

3:00 pm   **Break**

3:15 pm   **Session 4: Innovative Technologies, Tools, and Strategies
to Support the Cancer Careforce**
Moderator: Ruth Nemire, American Association of
Colleges of Pharmacy

- **Trends in technology and implications for the
careforce and cancer care**
Mia Levy, Rush University Cancer Center

- **Highlighting effective and promising approaches
to support the cancer careforce (5-minute lightning
presentations)**
  o **Family caregiving and advanced practice providers**
Kathi Mooney, The University of Utah
  o **Chat bot using artificial intelligence**
Samuel Takvorian, University of Pennsylvania

- o **Project ECHO**
    Kathleen Schmeler, The University of Texas
        MD Anderson Cancer Center
- o **Scribes**
    Eben Rosenthal, Stanford Comprehensive Cancer
        Center
- o **eConsults**
    Scott Shipman, Association of American Medical
        Colleges
- o **Technology + people for patient navigation**
    Hugh Ma, RobinCare, Inc.
- o **Goals of care conversations initiative**
    Jill Lowery, Department of Veterans Affairs and
        Duke University

Panel Discussion

5:30 pm   Adjourn Day 1

5:35 pm   Reception

February 12, 2019

7:30 am   Registration and Breakfast

**8:00 am   Session 5: Opportunities to Scale and Spread Solutions
               to Address Careforce Challenges**
               Moderator: Robert Carlson, National Comprehensive
                   Cancer Network

**How can we more effectively and efficiently disseminate
innovations to address careforce needs on a national
level?**

- • **Payment and health insurance**
    Harold Paz, Aetna

- • **Leveraging organizational culture and leadership to
    promote change**
    Howard "Skip" Burris, Sarah Cannon Research
        Institute

- **What disruptive innovations could change the delivery of cancer care and spur progress in better supporting the careforce?**
  Susan Dentzer, Duke University

Panel Discussion

9:30 am   **Break**

9:45 am   **Session 6: Stakeholder Recommendations on a Policy Agenda and Framework for Action**
Moderator: Lisa Kennedy Sheldon, Oncology Nursing Society

Panelists
- Brenda Nevidjon, Oncology Nursing Society
- Hildy Dillon, Cancer Support Community
- Courtney Van Houtven, Duke University and Department of Veterans Affairs
- John Cox, University of Texas Southwestern Medical Center
- Ronald Kline, Centers for Medicare & Medicaid Services
- Randall Oyer, Penn Medicine Lancaster General Health and the Association of Community Cancer Centers
- Mark Hyde, Huntsman Cancer Institute
- Ruth Nemire, American Association of Colleges of Pharmacy

11:30 am   **Workshop Wrap-Up**
Lisa Kennedy Sheldon, Oncology Nursing Society
Lawrence Shulman, University of Pennsylvania
Planning Committee Co-Chairs

11:45 am   **Adjourn**